LIFTOFF

COUCH TO BARBELL

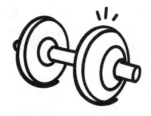

CASEY JOHNSTON

LIFTOFF: Couch to Barbell
Second edition
Copyright © 2024 by She's A Beast LLC
All rights reserved.
ISBN: 979-8-218-52289-6

No part of this publication may be reproduced, stored in a retrieval system, or transmitted in a form by means electronic, mechanical, photocopied, recorded, or otherwise, without the prior written consent of the publisher.

The authors and publisher disclaims any responsibility for any adverse effects or consequences from the misapplication or injudicious use of the information presented in this text.

Published October 15, 2024

Email: support@couchtobarbell.com
Website: couchtobarbell.com
#couchtobarbell

DISCLAIMER

This book is not intended for the treatment or prevention of disease or injury, and is not a substitute for, nor an alternative to, medical advice.

Look: I am excited for everyone to try lifting. Nothing makes me feel like I could squat 900 pounds like someone telling me they tried lifting heavy weights and now everything in their life is different.

But in putting out a program for beginners, I have to consider the other side of the coin, which is that I would be devastated if even a single person hurt themselves badly trying out this program. I have tried to make something that starts slow and is maximally accessible, but not everything can work for everyone.

Therefore, no one should follow this program who has a medical condition or chronic illness that contraindicates exercising or strength training. If there is any reasonable doubt in your mind about your personal health, please visit a doctor or your favorite medical professional to get the all-clear before doing this, or anything like this. I'm not saying this to get in your way or discourage anyone, and there's risk involved in everything we do. But I don't accept that this should be a high-stakes dangerous journey for anyone. Use of this book is at the choice and risk of the reader alone.

I want strength for all of us, but nothing is worth getting badly hurt. Don't be a hero.

CONTENTS

The quick and dirty spiritual rules of LIFTOFF 1
How to use this guide and spreadsheet 3
Introduction 7
Why should I learn to lift? The goals of LIFTOFF 13
Who is this program for? 19
Free weights, compound movements,
   and why they matter 27
What's going to happen to your body 31
Program structure 43
The lifts 47
Weights go up 55
Warming up 59
General cues, breathing, and the singular joy of a rep 63
Phase One 69
Phase Two 89
Phase Three 113
When to go to a gym 129
How to start going to the gym 137
Recording your workouts 149

Failing, and getting a spotter 153
Recovery, or "eating and resting" 155
What to do if you stall (and a note about OHP) 165
A note on deadlifts 169
A note on squat depth 173
What's next 177
FAQs 183
Further considerations 197
Appendix A: Terms 201
Appendix B: Liftoff Phases One, Two,
    and Three templates 217
Credits/sources 229
Resources 231

THE QUICK AND DIRTY SPIRITUAL RULES OF LIFTOFF

This is about skills. LIFTOFF is a 12-week, skill-building, strength-building program. It is not a weight loss program. It is not a "no mercy 'til you're pouring sweat and your vision blurs" program. If you only want to "work up a sweat" or "burn calories," go elsewhere. These things may happen here, but they are not the point!

You live in your body; make it nice. LIFTOFF is a functional strength training program, which means both that 1) the selected movements mirror the ways your body is built to move, and 2) the strength they build will translate extremely well to the pushing, pulling, carrying, and picking up that you do in real life.

Weights go up. You are here to build strength and skills. To do that, you have to make progress. Progress is what almost every "weight lifting" program you've ever tried was probably missing. LIFTOFF uses a "weights go up" system, where you add a small and sustainable amount of weight to each lift every session. In order to make that happen, you need to challenge yourself appropriately—not too hard, but not too easy either. You also need to take care of yourself, which brings us to...

Recovery matters. Building strength is part of a harmonious cycle. What you do outside of the gym is as important as what you do inside. Eating well and resting well means you train well. We hold these truths to be self-evident: You have to eat. You have to sleep. You have to tell energy vampires to fuck off, and sources of stress to stand down. For the next 12 weeks, you are busy getting stronger.

Form matters. The lifts in LIFTOFF use whole muscle systems; it's why they are called "compound lifts." We are naturally good at them, but our bodies learn a lot of less-than-helpful compensations to get along in modern life (bending over at the waist because pants are too restrictive to bend our knees and hips, for instance). These moves are worth learning to do with good form because they mimic real-life movement, AND keep our workouts mercifully short. Good form is a journey, not a destination.

Say hello, to yourself. A huge part of LIFTOFF is learning about your body. What does "good and challenging" versus "bad and too hard" feel like? What mental cues help you deadlift best? How many and which foods help your training go well? What feels scary to you in particular that you need to break down into smaller steps? Uncertainty and new things can be intimidating. But learning to be generous to yourself as you learn a new activity is core to what makes LIFTOFF rewarding.

BEFORE YOU CONTINUE
HOW TO USE THIS BOOK

LIFTOFF: Couch to Barbell (this book) has everything you need to get started with lifting. This book contains some instruction for the lifting movements themselves, but they are admittedly complicated to explain in words. That is why, at the time I created this program, I also created instructional videos for each of the lifts, which you are encouraged to watch and follow along as much as needed. You can find these videos at couchtobarbell.com/videos, sorted by Phase. There are also additional lists of videos from other trusted sources at the bottom of each page.

At the end of this book are the program templates for Phases One, Two, and Three, which you are encouraged to copy into a notebook of your choice. You don't need to reproduce the exact format; you just want to be able to keep track of what weights you lifted, how many times, each day. Tracking your progress is a very important part of lifting!

At the end of the book, you will also find formulas for warm-up set weights, and a formula for your Total Daily Energy Expenditure and protein intake for when you are linearly progressing your weights by lifting three times per week (both of these will be explained in following sections).

This program is designed so that you can hop into training right away with Phase One, which consists of bodyweight movements only (instructions covered in the related instructional videos). You **do not** need to read this book beginning to end in order to get started.

If you want to better understand why lifting is for you, I strongly recommend reading the "Why should I learn to lift?" and "Who is this program for" sections.

While you start moving through Phase One, you have time to take in some of the other aspects of the program, including:

- Why we use free weights
- The program structure
- What the deal is with all the lifts
- General cues
- How to warm up
- Why "weights go up" matters
- Why and how to record your lifts and progress
- How to pick weights
- Why failing matters
- What you should (or shouldn't) be doing other than lifting

How to eat, rest, and recover to support your training

I recommend being ready to take your eating and resting seriously by the time you head into Phase Two. You should be mentally prepared to eat enough protein, and have made your peace with not focusing on "burning calories" and "losing weight." You don't have to have everything down perfectly! But "weights go up" doesn't happen without taking care of yourself.

You can read each Phase Two and Phase Three section as you approach them, and you can watch the related form videos accordingly. Phase One is when you may start to encounter issues with squat depth; Phase Two is when you may begin to encounter stalling and overhead press problems; Phase Three is when you might have to negotiate your deadlift setup a little bit. There are special sections toward the end of the book for all of these issues. **Any of the Phases can be extended or shortened to your liking, depending on your level of progress physically or emotionally.**

A big part of this project is helping people see how gratifying and rewarding strength training can be; that it's not just for elites lifting a thousand pounds; and that working out doesn't have to be about weight loss, frenetic activity, and guilt. If you're on that page, **share your journey with the hashtag #couchtobarbell**, mostly because I want to cheer you on, but also so you can find others who understand the experience you're having.

If you have issues, such as soreness, equipment availability, having to miss days of training, embarrassment, injury, or boredom: These are very normal problems! Refer to the FAQ. If you don't know any of the words or terms being used, refer to the "Terms" section.

Once you've reached week 12 (or wherever you're at after a few weeks of using a barbell!) refer to the "What's next" section. The short answer is that, if you like the last phase of LIFTOFF, you can keep doing it until the weights you lift are no longer going up every session. If you don't like it or are done with it, you can stop and go do something else!

If you'd like to do even more reading about lifting beyond this book, my newsletter, She's A Beast, has covered an enormous range of topics and questions from readers just like you. You can access the entire archive at shesabeast.co.

If you have any questions or feedback, email: support@couchtobarbell.com

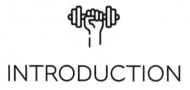

INTRODUCTION

WHERE AM I?

This is a strength training program for people who want to go from zero familiarity with lifting weights to comfortably and confidently lifting heavy weights, including a barbell. That's what makes it "couch to barbell."

This program will take you from learning the bodyweight versions of several different lifting movements; on through the dumbbell versions of the movements; and finally, to the barbell versions of these movements. Once you are finished with this program, you will be able to lift 45 pounds, and probably more, in several different ways. You will also feel and see all the physical changes that come with learning that skill!

WHY CALL IT 'LIFTOFF'?

In the gym, a "liftoff" is when a fellow bro stands above/behind you when you are benching and helps you lift the barbell out of the rack, and positions it over your shoulders so you can start your rep. It's strong people helping strong people. It's what I hope to do for you, metaphorically: Help get you into position to build your own strength.

"Liftoff" in the space travel sense is also a nice metaphor. You'll be going from zero to breaking through the atmosphere that has contained you for so long.

I also really like the song "Liftoff" by Jay Z and Kanye West feat. Beyoncé. If I had my way, it would play every time I thought or spoke about LIFTOFF, but alas, rights conspire to keep us apart.

WHO ARE YOU, CASEY JOHNSTON/A SWOLE WOMAN?

To run through my background very quickly: I was crushed under the pressure of dieting and being thin, beginning in high school. To support my desire to constantly lose weight, I took up long-term crash dieting and cardio. At first I dragged myself through 15 minutes of running three times a week, and I stopped to walk... a lot. Then I was running three miles at a time, then five, then six, then nine, then 13. I ran four half-marathons by 2014 before I realized that all this running wasn't getting me fucking anywhere, emotionally or physically.

But then lifting started to get kind of cool, and all kinds of people were posting about it online: about how it made them feel (extremely good) what it made them look like (pretty awesome actually), how much stronger they were able to get (a lot pretty easily), how much time they actually had to spend in the gym (not much), and how much they ate in order for the overall process to work (a lot). In 2014 I dove in to a book, Mark Rippetoe's *Starting Strength*, and never looked back.

Well, except I did look back. The problem with *Starting Strength* was that it assumed its readers are already strong enough to handle at least a 45lb barbell. When I started lifting, I couldn't even pick up a barbell to *move* it, much less squat it. And yet every beginner resource I could find required both knowing what a barbell was and being able to lift one already.

This led to a lot of bouncing back and forth between the book and various other increasingly arcane online resources. I had to kind of carve my own path to actually being able to use a barbell by picking through dozens of different spreadsheets, form videos, and programs. But I quickly became bonkers for strength training. Once I learned to do it, I could not shut up about how incredible and transformative it was, how good it felt, and how my relationship with my body and with food were finally good and made sense to me.

All the research I had to do to get started would have been a lot to ask of a regular person who just wants to get a little strong, and doesn't want to have to learn everything there is to know about strength training theory and practice. I also had fears about what lifting would "do" to me, and felt intimidated overall by the process; I could have used more reassurance about that.

I got to a point where I loved strength training so much that I wanted to help others get over these emotional and logistical humps. So five years ago, I started writing a column for The Hairpin called Ask A Swole Woman to help people understand that strength training, and the lifestyle it entails, is suited to far, far more people than the stereotypical macho guy we picture in a weight room. With LIFTOFF, I'm synthesizing the philosophy and practical advice of many of those columns into one comprehensive guide to how, as well as why, everyone can and should try strength training.

LIFTOFF: Couch to Barbell is the thing I wish had existed when I first got interested in lifting: a program and guide that would first allow me to get comfortable with the basic compound movements in my own home; then progress me to using small weights at home or in a gym; and finally, transition me to using a barbell.

I made LIFTOFF because I think everyone can learn something from lifting weights. Lifting weights isn't just about raw strength, and it's not just for the people who are pre-ordained to be strong. It's also about having a constructive, positive-feedback-loop relationship with your body. It's about mobility; body mechanics; and managing, or even heading off, the pain we may experience from moving too little in the ways we are naturally good at. And, okay, it's also about how fucking good it feels to be strong.

You may notice there is not a ton of actual "lifting instruction" in this book. That is because all of that is more quickly, and more simply, explained by the videos linked in the appropriate places (plus, it's easier to quickly pull up a short video between sets in the gym than it is to flip to the right page and read a bunch of text). This book covers everything else: why LIFTOFF contains the movements it does and why it's structured the way it is; what you can expect to get out of it; how to approach the three phases; how to progress; how to fail; how to take care of yourself outside the gym; how to deal with stalling; and a long, comprehensive explainer on how to progress with deadlifts when you can't (yet) set the barbell up at the right height. There is also a long FAQs section, and a less-long "terms" section.

You may be thinking: How simple can this really be, if this book is so long? My friend—I can't tell you how many hours, days, weeks, *months* I spent poring over little fitness influencer workouts, trying to learn them, feeling embarrassed by them, and giving up on them. I can't tell you how much time I spent thinking "exercise" and "food" were only and exclusively meant to be manipulated around "losing weight," because that's how they were presented to me pretty much everywhere. This is to say nothing of all the time I spent anxiously studying celebrity photos and interviews, trying to reverse engineer what makes them so fit, and only ending up in a 1,200-calories-and-"core training" prison of my own design.

All those hours amount to far, far less time than it will take you to read this book. I sort of hope this is the last workout you will every really have to learn how to do, because these skills can and will serve you forever, if you let them. It's also a perfect basis for learning everything *else* there is to know about lifting weights, as I will explain.

WHY SHOULD I LEARN TO LIFT?

THE GOALS OF LIFTOFF

Why do all of this? More importantly, why read all of this? A few reasons:

As someone who used to have an extremely impoverished relationship with my body and food, lifting changed all of that for me 180 degrees. I didn't realize that I didn't need to be a bodybuilder in order to enjoy and benefit from a short-term cycle of strength training.

Lifting is for everyone, and it's especially for anyone who has never done any strength training before, and it's especially *especially* for everyone who has been trapped in cycles of dieting and weight loss for years and years of their existence (see the "What's going to happen to your body" section for more on this).

The best thing of all about strength training is that once you build strength, you have it, to a certain extent, forever. Thanks to muscle memory, when we do some strength training, we always keep some abilities and physical adaptations which will allow us to:

1. Stay strong with less effort than it took to get strong in the first place. We need muscle for our health, but we also need it for making our daily lives feel good. This also means it pays off across all other activities—dancing, yoga, cycling, running, bringing the latest box delivered to your doorstep inside.
2. Get strong again with less effort than it took the first time, if we were to give up strength training for a while and then return to it later. Yes, this is really just how bodies work!

INTENSITY AND TRAINING VS. WORKOUTS, EXPLAINED

Lifting weights is the best expression I've ever found of the positive feedback loop that can exist between training, fueling ourselves and feeling good. But none of us know about this part of lifting, because strength training is all wrapped up in weird cultural stereotypes. Many fitness personalities selling their little jumpy-up-and-downy, tiny-pulses, resistance-band-filled programs are stoking our outsize fears about "bulkiness," or feeding our worries that it's not feminine, or refined, or cerebral to lift big weights.

Because we are so focused on *workouts*, not *training*, exercise can feel like a never-ending, lifelong slog: We feel like we can only stay thin if we keep running mile after mile after mile, if we keep subscribing to Kayla Itsines' SWEAT app, if we keep alerts on for Ally Love's Peloton classes. But with slightly more structure, and by thinking of exercise in terms of training instead of as one-off workouts, the whole activity can gain a new meaning.

When you "exercise," you might go "as hard as you possibly can" for 5 or 10 or 20 minutes doing various movements. This is not strength training, no matter what the New York Times or any TikTok influencer calls it. The difference between *a workout* and *training* is smart, predictable increase of intensity (or, as we will cover shortly, "weights go up"). Intensity doesn't mean "harder," and it doesn't mean "a bigger, longer, or more painful grind." In lifting, more intensity can mean only that the weights go up, but the reps stay on the low side (for instance, 35 pounds for 5 reps is more intense than 10 pounds for 20 reps). This measured intensity in training is what allows strength to grow. When you are *training*, you squat 40 pounds for 5 sets of 5 reps today, then 45 pounds for 5 sets of 5 reps at the next squat session, and so on.

Intensity doesn't necessarily mean "more difficulty," because you only ever push yourself according to *your* current capacity to get stronger. More intensity does not mean you sweat more, or hurt more, the next day (in fact, you will probably sweat and hurt less than when you do the average YouTube fitness influencer workout). But bodies are good at getting stronger and growing a little under these moderately-more-intense conditions; it's just harder to explain this than it is to say "do chair dips for 45 seconds," which is why many workouts just tell you to do chair dips for 45 seconds.

Training also means you eat and rest to support your time in the gym to ensure you'll be able to make "weights go up" next time. By doing all this, you can build strength that is yours, and will stay yours, forever.

The aim of this program is that, by the time you complete Phase Three, you will be able to confidently handle a

45lb barbell, and then some. From there, whole worlds of strength training, functional fitness, hypertrophy, bodybuilding, and butt building are all unlocked to you, if you want. Technically, you can do all of this stuff without being strong, but the effects of any weight training program are greatly enhanced by having a "strength base," a fundamental amount of neurological and muscular strength. That's what LIFTOFF is designed to build. And if all you want is to be able to maintain a bit of strength with other kinds of workouts, that will be unlocked for you, too.

While the practical goal of this program is building a strength base, I hope that in the process you will also learn about yourself, and gain more empathy for yourself, more resiliency, and a more expansive definition of "who" you "are." It's corny, but strength training teaches you to grow, and when you are someone who can grow, you can become anything.

THE HARD NUMBERS

In more brass-tacks terms, you might be wondering where you're going to end up, in terms of numbers. There are no hard-and-fast results statistics you are trying to hit; you are strongly encouraged to progress in the weights you lift, but also to learn to pay attention to how you feel and dial in what's right for you.

This is covered more in the "Weights go up" section, but let's just do some ballpark figures.

"Add at least 2.5lbs to all my upper body lifts, and 5lbs to my lower body lifts every session for 12 weeks" is the target progress pace for "weights go up." This means that if you start from absolute zero and progress steadily, your numbers at the end of the program would look like this:

Squat: 75 pounds (barbell + 30lbs)
Deadlift: 75 pounds
Overhead press: 37.5 pounds
Bench: 37.5 pounds
Row: 37.5 pounds
Lat pulldown: 37.5 pounds

If you started each lift able at 10-20 pounds, it would look like this:

Squat: 95 pounds (barbell + 50lbs)
Deadlift: 95 pounds
Overhead press: 47.5 pounds (barbell + 2.5lbs)
Bench: 47.5 pounds
Row: 47.5 pounds
Lat pulldown: 47.5 pounds

If you started with 10-20 pounds, and instead went up by 5-10lbs per session, it would look like this:

Squat: 160 pounds (barbell + 115lbs)
Deadlift: 160 pounds
Overhead press: 80 pounds (barbell + 35lbs)
Bench: 80 pounds
Row: 80 pounds
Lat pulldown: 80 pounds

Most likely, you will end up somewhere in the middle of the second and third position. You might even end up with higher numbers! That's okay. If you feel afraid to add 5 or 10lbs to a lift, I would suggest trying it every once in a while. Definitely use your first session to experiment a bit and find the right starting place for you.

Maybe these numbers sound low to you. You can move as fast as you want, and also, technically, keep going with strength training as long as you want. I'm just here to bridge the gap between "zero" and "barbell."

Maybe these numbers sound high to you, to the point of being impossible. I swear on my own meticulously kept Ohio Power Bar, lifting weights is obviously not no effort at all, but it IS going to be much easier than you think. If you make the appointment to meet yourself at the gym, planning to lift 5 pounds more than last time, having eaten your protein and gotten your sleep, you will be there.

WHO IS THIS PROGRAM FOR?

This program is for anyone who feels alienated by the burden of their physical self and their body that's never hot enough, always in too much pain, and never able to show up when it counts, like when you have to bring groceries in from the car, or simply move a 40lb box of cat litter, or rearrange the furniture in the living room. "I really should work out," we say to ourselves in these moments. And then we do an Orange Theory class, or a follow-along HIIT workout on YouTube, and those things don't really seem to change much for us in terms of "feeling different" except "maybe a little less winded when you take the stairs."

Our workouts can, and should, do more than this, without requiring significantly more effort. LIFTOFF will do more than this for you.

This program is also for people for whom exercise has never really... clicked. Maybe nothing you've ever done has felt worth the shame/embarrassment/sweat you're trading away, and at best workouts feel like varying degrees of torture, supposedly in service of "being hot" and "losing weight." Maybe those goals were exciting at first, but quickly lost their sheen as the path between "going to [insert activity] class several times a week" and "the #bodygoals you were sold by the marketing for that class" became fuzzier and fuzzier.

This can happen because we have misplaced so much of what working out can be about—understanding our bodies as nice places to live; as functional tools; as giving us a measured sense of achievement; as creating a positive feedback loop along with the ways we eat and rest. For decades, we have been glossing over all of that, in favor of making it entirely about being hot and "losing weight" (especially when we say we want to "lose weight," when what we really mean is that we want to "change our body composition"; see the "What's going to happen to your body" for more on this).

Let me be abundantly clear: I am here neither to try and make you conventionally hot, nor to make you lose weight, nor sweat, nor "burn calories" (though those things may happen!).

This is not to say I think people are bad for ever wanting these things. But the singular focus on weight loss has turned food and exercise into a guilt-driven and complicated circus, when they should be just basic ways that we take care of ourselves. Many things about focusing on weight loss not only don't work for most of us, but become a compounding problem. We crash-diet to lose weight, and end up losing muscle along the way; we regain the weight, mostly as body fat, because the way we lost the weight was not a sustainable lifestyle; and repeat, until a lot of our muscle is gone, undermining our metabolism and ability to feel good in our bodies. This is the Avocado Principle at work (more about this in the "What's going to happen to your body" section).

Dieting too much and feeling pressure to work out a lot are discordant forms of torture. Working out, and strength training in particular, can be an entirely different journey separate from these things. Eating for joy and to make working out feel good, and training to feel good in your body, can be harmonious. If you are into harmony and not discord, then this all might just be right for you.

I don't promise to change your whole life. But I do promise to deliver skills—that is, how to move and take care of yourself while you learn to do that—and a feeling, which is that your body can be a nicer place to be and less of the enemy you think it is. The point is to see yourself get stronger, to learn basic movement skills, and to see the lifestyle benefits that lifting creates: mobility, capability, a constructive relationship with your body and food.

If you've never understood the right way to bend down and pick something up "using your legs and not your back," this is for you. If you are afraid of squatting all the way down because it might hurt your knees, this is for you. If your body generally hurts and feels stiff from sitting too much, this is for you.

This is also for you if you've been curious about lifting weights, or have heard that "strength training is essential" for some other goal that resonates with you, but you feel like a total ignoramus about how to get started. You might not even know what a barbell is; maybe you've never even worked up the nerve to set foot in the weight room; maybe you don't know a deadlift from a forklift or an overhead press from a panini press. That's extremely okay; you are "most people."

If you've ever attempted to get into strength training, you might have noticed that most beginner programs fall into two categories: They completely avoid heavy weights, tend to focus on little bodyweight movements, and have a goal of "weight loss or "toning"; or, they are for people who can already easily handle a barbell and have been lifting so long they need "17 New Moves for Back Day" to keep the relationship alive. You might have even tried the former and been surprised and disappointed by either its difficulty or lack of results, and were probably too intimidated or felt too incompetent to try the latter.

In my day, wannabe lifters who couldn't yet handle a barbell were left to piece together how to get to the level of strength necessary for "real" weight training. Many "strength training" or "weight training" programs may use weights, but don't give us any scheme to progress with. This makes them more like just workouts than transformative skill-building. In contrast, this guide bridges the gap between "never done this before" and "can handle a barbell with ease and confidence."

This program is unique in that it will guide you from absolutely zero familiarity with lifting weights, through low-stakes bodyweight versions of functional movements, to dumbbell versions of these movements, and finally into the barbell versions of these movements. You will get stronger steadily and predictably, and gain the skill of "being able to move heavy things."

WHAT IF I ALREADY DO A SPORT?

In all my years of talking with people about lifting, I've found a fair number of folks who are interested in lifting weights, and even are already habitual exercisers or are passionate about a sport, but they shy away from lifting for one reason or another. Often that reason is that all of the lifting content out there feels like they need to make a whole new and permanent lifestyle change, and possibly even give up their sport in order to live the life of a meathead. This is not the case.

All kinds of weight training begin with the same phase: building a "strength base." Bodybuilders do it, powerlifters do it, and athletes do it. When you build a strength base, you steadily ramp up your muscles' capability, which lays the foundation for making almost any other kind of training more effective.

A bodybuilder who wants to have massive biceps won't get very massive biceps if he can only curl 15 pounds. But if that bodybuilder puts in a few months of benching and rowing to lay his strength base, soon he might be able to curl 40 pounds. Now he is getting somewhere.

Likewise, a rock climber might love rock climbing, but find that their ability to do harder routes is limited by their leg weakness when they try to rock over. If that rock climber put in a few months of basic squats and deadlifts, their fundamental strength would be much less of a limiting factor; they still need to practice technique, but they are working from a better, stronger foundation.

We often make the mistake that people are good at the sports they do only because they do those specific sports a lot. But this is also not the case. Boxers don't punch hard, soccer players don't fire in shots on goal, and gymnasts don't launch themselves into the air without being pretty dang strong. And we often don't see the training that goes into that. But it's common for athletes to work on this kind of strength separately from practicing their sport. You can do this, too.

Even if you are not sure if strength training is for you in the long run, you might recognize that giving a temporary, primary focus to strength training would enrich your enjoyment of other activities. LIFTOFF is designed as a complete strength-foundation-building phase to fill in that part of your athletic background. The program asks that you scale back the other workouts or training you are passionate about, but only for a set period of time. You're not changing your identity. You don't have to mold yourself anew in the image of Arnold Schwarzenegger or Kayla Itsines. You're doing something that will support all of your other activities, whether that is carrying groceries, doing a viral TikTok challenge, or learning to do a death-drop in pole dancing.

There are "strength training" workouts out there meant to be integrated into, say, a half-marathon training program to build complementary stability or endurance instead of meaningful strength (particularly because your body needs rest as part of building strength, and you won't get much rest while training for a half marathon). LIFTOFF is not that.

LIFTOFF is designed as a minimum effective dose of strength training for beginners. It is hard to produce strength and functionality doing either a lot less or a lot more than this. It may not look like what you are used to! Often, strength training programs we see are very complex, and that's because they are designed for more advanced users. People who are just starting out can take a much simpler, minimalist approach, and see a consistent, rewarding payoff.

WHO ISN'T THIS PROGRAM FOR?

Some caveats: this is a program for people who aren't afraid of challenging themselves, who want to create transformative change in the way they move. If you don't yet know what "pushing yourself" looks or feels like, I want you to be open to experimenting and finding out.

If you just want to "get a bit of a sweat going" or "burn calories" and aren't interested in how your body works, or in changing your body composition after too many years of dieting, or in feeling appreciably stronger, there is tonnnns of stuff on YouTube et al. for you. LIFTOFF is not everything to everyone, and that's by design.

This program is not for people who can only be satisfied by a lot of frenetic activity or variety. I love strength training because it's a universe in a grain of sand; squats are relatively easy to learn, but you can spend a lifetime perfecting them. The interesting part, to me, is learning to help your body move in a functional way.

This program is also not for people who can't accept that strength is only built slowly with consistent, high-intensity effort (bearing in mind that "high intensity" is not the same as "extreme difficulty"). It's not a high-rep, low-weight program (if anything, it's the opposite), and it's not a body-weight program. It's not for people who are going to let their unfounded fear of "being bulky," or their desire to "only be toned," override and sabotage their progress in this program.

Gender, body type, training background, and age do not matter here (though for reasons of my liability, please be over 18 and in good, medical-professional-certified health). If you would like to learn to be strong, this is the program to do it.

FREE WEIGHTS, COMPOUND MOVEMENTS, AND WHY THEY MATTER

The LIFTOFF program is made up of "compound movements." The first Google result describes compound movements as "multi-joint movements that work several muscles or muscle groups at one time," and that's pretty dang spot-on.

If you are like I was before I started lifting, you probably understand "lifting weights" as "using all of the various machines in the gym to work one muscle at a time." If you wanted to work out your legs, you'd use the knee extension machine; then the hamstring curl machine; then hip abductor machine; then the leg press machine, then the calf raise machine. This takes, conservatively, eighty dozen sets and four million reps.

I was not aware that machines are actually more niche than they seem, given how much space they take up in gyms. Weights built into a machine move on gliding tracks and "target" muscles, more so for size than anything (they are perfect for bodybuilders trying to bulk up that one part of their leg).

But in the real world, the stuff we have to move and pick up and carry around, including our own body parts, are not perfectly secured in a gliding track. We also don't move around in the world the way that machines train us, by separately first moving our glutes, then our adductors, then our hamstrings, then our quads. Instead, we stand up. We take a step forward. We pick things up. We push things around. Our muscles are fundamentally good at working together, if we just give them a chance. Machines are not for people who are trying to build holistic physical capability, who want to "move better" and hurt less and be in shape. In the grand scheme of training, they are side dishes, not the main course.

So what is a person who wants to move better and hurt less and be in shape to do? That's where compound movements with free weights come in. Free weights used in compound movements, like squats or deadlifts or bench, are designed around how your body's muscles are meant to work together. Not only do compound movements have the benefit of being "what your body is already good at," you can get strong at them much faster than working each individual muscle at a time, and this makes workouts way shorter. In LIFTOFF, instead of the aforementioned 17 machines and eighty dozen sets and four million reps, you would do 5 sets of 5 squats, and that's it.

Is that all there is to working out for the rest of your life? Maybe not. But compound movements should very likely always be the centerpiece of a functional workout meant to build your strength base, and at least for the duration of LIFTOFF, that's all there is to it.

In LIFTOFF we do compound movements with free weights like barbells and dumbbells. Using free weights lets our bodies learn to stabilize themselves when we are under tension. And unlike with machines targeting one individual muscle at a time, it's very difficult to train these little stabilizer muscles in concert with all your other muscles. That's why it's important to put your body in a situation where it can move freely, the way it is when you move things in real life.

Still skeptical? What if I told you stabilizers included "your core," and that you'll be working your core throughout most of your workout thanks to using free weights? Oh yeah, baby; now I bet I have your attention. After all, what matters more in our society than having a "strong core"?

If all that doesn't convince you, this should: Compound movements are not inherently more difficult, and by using more muscles at once, they save time. Truly! You can do 3 sets each of chest flyes, tricep machine, curl machine, lateral raise machine, front raise machine; OR, you can bench 45 pounds for 3 sets of 5 reps, and then go home. Which one do you have the time and patience for?

WHAT'S GOING TO HAPPEN TO YOUR BODY

Muscle is the best kind of body mass there is (I guess apart from your vital organs), and it basically can never hurt to have a little more. Muscle helps with metabolism, protects you from injury, and allows you to move well overall.

A little muscle goes a long way. But a little muscle is easy to lose. It can happen by dieting for long periods of time, or in repeated, aggressive cycles. I call this, plus the related processes of building muscle and body recomposition, the Avocado Principle.

These are some diagrams to explain, in very simple terms, what happens to your body composition when you diet too aggressively for too long, using an avocado as a visual analogy (the "pit" is your lean body mass, while the green part is body fat):

"LOSING WEIGHT"
(TRYING TO GET SMALLER, REGARDLESS OF WHAT IS LOST; BAD)

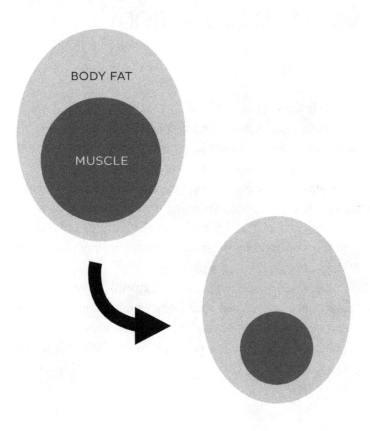

► Up to half of weight lost can be muscle, if you"re too harsh.

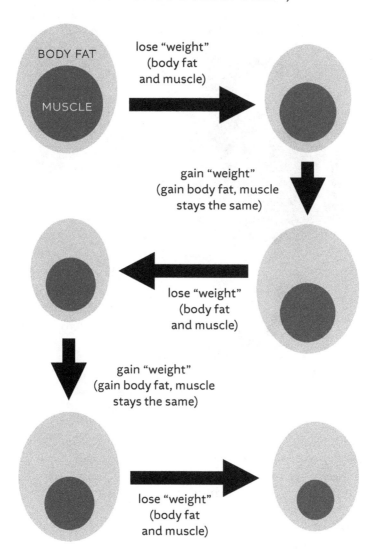

"YO YO DIETING" THE SHORT VERSION

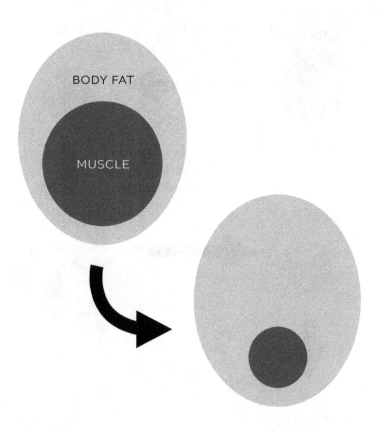

▸ Same weight, roughly same size, muscle has gone bye bye

Muscle likewise takes deliberate effort and time to gain back, but doing so can help reverse the damage done to muscle mass by dieting too much. When you lift weights, assuming you hold your maintenance calories (see the "Recovery" section) and body weight constant, your body will lose some body fat and gain some muscle. This means, while the weight on the scale doesn't change, you may begin to see slightly more definition, and your clothes may fit a little looser. This is what that looks like:

"RECOMPOSITION"
(BUILDING MUSCLE AND LOSING BODY FAT AT THE SAME TIME)

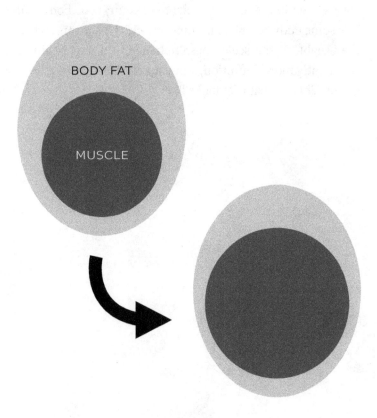

- Body about same size or slightly smaller (muscle weighs more than fat.
- Weight about the same.

And in the longer term, it's possible to keep building muscle without ultimately changing body size very much:

BUILDING MUSCLE
THE LONG VERSION

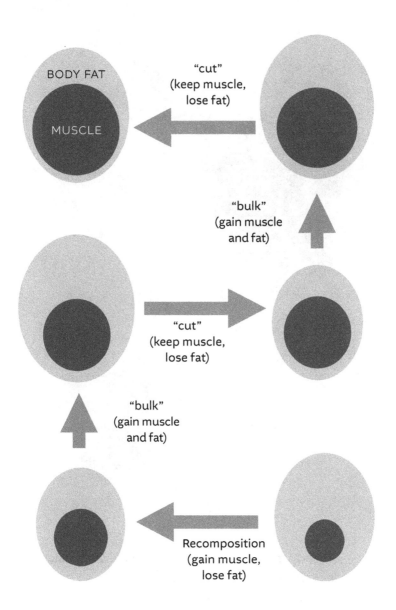

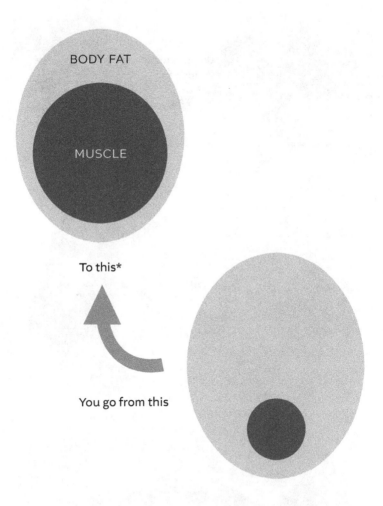

Even building 10 pounds of muscle, for most women, is probably close to two years' worth of work (for men, it's about a year). If you gained two or three pounds of muscle total during LIFTOFF, that would be considered "crazy amazing" results. You will see that that's not a night and day difference, but you may notice some small changes. That is why aesthetic changes are not the goal of LIFTOFF; if they were, you would probably be disappointed.

But a program like LIFTOFF sets you up incredibly well if you do aim to change your body composition a lot and later want to do bodybuilding, or continue recomposition (losing body fat and/or gaining muscle). There is no realm in which building strength and muscle won't ultimately help with body composition changes, if that is your goal.

HOW DO MUSCLES GROW?

You may have been disappointed in the past that lifting two-pound dumbbells for lots and lots of reps did not ever really do anything for you. You may have also heard that lifting heavy, challenging-for-you weights for relatively fewer reps is what creates actual strength and muscle. Let me explain this a little more.

Here is a thought experiment: Picture a sheet of paper, and imagine crumpling and uncrumpling it. After a lot of crumplings and uncrumplings, it is a little more ragged than before. This is like what cardio (or lifting tiny dumbbells for lots of reps) does to your muscles. If you were to try to "repair" the paper, the overall damage to it is pretty minor, and because it wasn't really harmed, there's not really room to make significant changes to the paper.

Now picture taking a different piece of paper and poking some big holes in it with a pencil. The paper is pretty mangled now, and you probably didn't even need to poke it that many times to absolutely thrash it, worse than anything lots of crumpling could do. The hole-poking is more like how lifting works on your muscles.

Now if you were to repair this second piece of paper, there are much bigger "opportunities" to "rebuild" it. The paper might even have so many holes, such large holes, that you can fit "more," and possibly "better," repair-paper into that space than there was before (we're gonna assume for the purposes of this thought experiment that the papers can be seamlessly fused together without you needing any particular skill). You started off with a flimsy sheet of copy paper, but now you're filling in the gaps with some thick and juicy cardstock. At the end, you actually have a slightly larger and more resilient piece of paper. This is, broadly, the difference between "cardio" and what is called "hypertrophy," which is what happens when you lift heavy weights. Bear in mind that even still, this process is incredibly slow. Even if you try as hard as you possibly can, building more than a few pounds of muscle takes years, not weeks.

A QUICK NOTE ON "BLOATING"

In the early phases of really any type of working out, including LIFTOFF, you may experience a bit of bloating or apparent "weight gain." This is normal; going from not working out to working out causes your body to kick into gear and retain more energy and water while it finds the equilibrium that works for your new energy demands.

Please be patient with this part. Lifting or working out is likely not "making you gain weight." Body weight and BMI are not amazing measures of health generally, and while totally uncoupling them is beyond the scope of LIFTOFF, please know that the point of LIFTOFF is not to make the number of pounds on the scale go down. It will likely not do that, but hopefully with what I've written so far, it's clear that that is not the way to measure success for a strength training program.

PROGRAM STRUCTURE

This program teaches you to lift in three phases:

Phase One is the Bodyweight Phase, with body weight/no weight versions of five basic movements. Every session is the same, three times a week.

Phase Two is the Dumbbell Phase, with movements that build on the movements from Phase One, but adding dumbbells. Instead of doing the same movements every day, Phase Two alternates two different days across three days each week, with the same basic movements spread out over those two days.

Phase Three is the Barbell Phase, with movements that build on the previous two phases, except now we're throwing a barbell in. By this time, you will have built enough strength to handle a 45lb empty barbell in some or all of the lifts.

This program never involves more than 5 sets, or more than 10 reps per set (and most movements are done for 3 to 5 sets of 5 reps). This is the minimum number of reps you can do to build strength as a beginner. As I've already said, we are not out here trying to do the most and run you ragged;

we are trying to build skills and strength. **This structure creates the conditions for building skills and strength, while minimizing the time that workouts take, as well as the number of trips needed to the gym, period.**

LIFTOFF is meant to be done three days a week, with at least one day of rest between workout days. Potential schedules that would fit here:

- Monday-Wednesday-Friday
- Tuesday-Thursday-Sunday
- Monday-Thursday-Saturday

You get the idea.

It's structured this way because, after breaking down your muscles, your body needs time to rest and recover and build your muscles back up better than they were before. To not take your rest days is to essentially mess up this process and waste your own time. See the "Recovery" section for more on this topic.

WHY IT'S SO "SIMPLE"

The best way to think of this program is "helping you understand your body and the value of building strength, at a minimum cost to you in terms of time and energy." This program is already a complete workout. Trainers will always be motivated to sell you increasingly complex or arcane programs out of insecurity or fear that they need to differentiate themselves from the one billion other trainers out there. They also do it because, if you can't complete a very complex and intense program with tons of reps and sets and therefore don't see results, whose fault is that? Complex programs help them, not you.

It will be very hard to do less than what LIFTOFF asks and expect to understand the transformative power of building strength, eating, and training. You can always do more, but I'm not here to help you do more. I'm here to help you understand the transformative power of lifting.

There will be a time when you can add in lots of accessory movements, or more complex rep schemes, or exciting variations of the basic movements. That time will be when these 12 weeks are over. If your temptation is to do way more on top of this already-taxing program, I think following this program would actually be a worthwhile experiment for you in learning to untangle "value" from "maximum effort possible at all times."

While some light activity on rest days can actually be helpful and not hurtful to a newbie lifter (see the 'What to do other than lifting' section), overdoing it will be hurtful. This is all a long way of saying, please don't paint outside the lines and then ask at the end why your picture doesn't look the way I promised.

A LITTLE MORE ABOUT THE STRUCTURE

LIFTOFF is unique because it flows from bodyweight movements, to dumbbell movements, and finally to barbell movements. It's made this way because your body is literally built to grow your strength and skills, and to adapt your muscles and neurons to the activities you do. Just as you can learn to run a 5K, you can learn to handle a barbell and then some.

LIFTOFF is designed to last 12 weeks with the suggested "weights go up" pace, but the length of each phase is more like a guideline; you can stay in each as long as you want or need to. For instance, if after five weeks of Phase Two, you aren't ready for any barbell movements, that's okay. You can keep repeating the alternating Phase Two sessions until you are. I only encourage eventually moving through all the phases.

LIFTOFF is a thoughtful combination of what we call "pushing" and "pulling" movements for both upper and lower body. These are the main building blocks of a strength training program. A squat is a push; a bench is a push; a deadlift is a pull; a lat pulldown is a pull. Most of what we do with our bodies is pushing and pulling. Running is a push; carrying groceries is a pull; picking up the box of cat litter is a pull; putting a suitcase into an overhead bin is a push.

Everything about the program, including the choice of movements; the order; and the number of sets and reps is deliberate, and optimized for balance and progress. If you want a program you can decoupage and Bedazzle with your own customizations, there are *tonnns* of other programs better suited to that. But LIFTOFF is designed to work as-is.

THE CORE LIFTS

To be clear, this book does not have extensive written instructions on how to do each compound lift; that kind of thing is much better suited to the videos linked within here. If a picture says a thousand words, a video says ten thousand. I'm trying to save you *some* reading.

That said, you might be curious why LIFTOFF uses these specific movements, so I'm going to explain briefly how they work and how they translate to your life. I'm doing this not for you to pick and choose; they're all meant to go together, and they all reinforce each other.

If any of the cues feel like too much to think about, just do your best to imitate what's happening in the videos, and refer here if your own form looks very off or the movement doesn't feel good.

SQUAT

This is probably the most familiar movement to you even if you've never stepped foot in a weight room, thanks to all those "bodyweight squat" challenges from a few years ago, or perhaps Megan Thee Stallion. In a squat, you bear weight near or on your shoulders or back; lower yourself down by bending at the hips and knees; and then come back up.

You might have noticed that life involves a lot of bending down. Squats will help enormously with this. They require a good bit of hip mobility in order to get your knees to track over your toes and prevent your butt from caving in at the bottom, all without your heels coming off the floor. You might not have this mobility when you first start. That's okay! Just the process of getting to the point where you have enough hip mobility to do a squat is going to be enormously valuable to you. Because of how we bear the weight in a free weight squat, squats are also great for building your "core stability."

Your squat should be deep enough that the crease your hip makes where it folds is below the top of your knee (this is called "below parallel"). Any higher than that is squatting "at" or "above parallel." Squatting to depth matters because your body uses different muscles once you reach below parallel, and it requires good, useful range of motion that squatting above parallel does not. See "A note on squat depth" if you struggle with this.

In this program, we begin with bodyweight squats, followed by dumbbell squats with the dumbbells racked on your shoulders, and finally move on to the barbell "high bar" squat.

"Cues" (form tips) to keep in mind:

- ▸ Heels shoulder width apart, heels stay on the ground, toes pointed out 30 degrees, weight in midfoot, barbell over midfoot (if applicable)
- ▸ Chest up, ribs down, core tight, knees track over toes
- ▸ Sit back in hips as you break at the knees, lower down until hip crease is below the very top of your knees
- ▸ It's okay if your knees go past your toes

BENCH

Benching is when you lie down on a bench, hold a weight above your chest, lower it until it touches your chest, and then press it back up. Benching makes any pushing activity you have to do easier—pushing furniture around, pushing a heavy grocery cart, pushing a heavy door closed.

Depending on your background, this might be one of the lifts you are most dreading, because it feels like it will involve competing for equipment with some of the biggest and/or bro-iest people in the gym. But easy there, grasshopper, we have a while yet until that happens. In this program, we build to barbell benching first with incline pushups (or regular push-ups, if you're able), followed by dumbbell bench press.

It can feel scary to hold weight over your body like this, but as with all the lifts, you aren't meant to do more than what is manageably challenging to you. A good bench set-up will also have "safety arms" on either side that will prevent the barbell from landing on you if it falls. When you get to the stage where failure is an actual risk, you can also ask one of the kind bros at the gym who love benching, and love to see other people bench, to spot you.

Bench cues to keep in mind:

- Move shoulders up, back, and down so the place your back is resting is situated toward the tops of your shoulder blades
- Weight stacked over your shoulders and wrists stacked over forearms (wrists should not bend back)
- Elbows at 45 degree angle to body
- Lower the bar to the bottom of your pecs/about where the bottom band of your bra sits

> Keeping elbows at the angle, press the weight back up without shifting shoulders out of position

DEADLIFT

"Deadlift" was a completely foreign term to me before I started lifting, but it refers to "lifting any 'dead' weight off the ground" (as opposed to a bench or squat, where the weight is "live" from the start of the lift, as it's supported by your body). In any deadlift, you are essentially bending down to grab any weight on the floor, and then standing up with it in your hands, in a way that is mechanically safe.

We do deadlifts because they are a highly functional movement, and translate extremely well to your real life. I don't know about you, but I'm picking stuff up from the ground and carrying it what feels like all of the time, and it used to be much more of a pain before I learned to deadlift.

In a barbell deadlift, you stand in front of a barbell on the floor with weight loaded on it, reach down to grab it with your hands, pack your body and legs down into position, and then stand up with the barbell in your hands. See, it's fun! This is really the part of the program where you learn to "lift with your legs, not your back" (which is not quite strictly true, but true enough).

Deadlifts are easy to grasp conceptually, but can be difficult to master. They require a bit more range of motion than you might think to get our bodies into position, and to do them without referring the entire lift to our lower backs. They also call upon our hip and leg muscles on the backs of our body, which can be pretty dormant for those of us who are mostly sedentary. That's okay; nothing will give them a wake-up call like a nice set of deadlifts. Also, fine: If you want to have a nice butt, I promise that nothing will set you up well for going on that journey like learning to do a nice, solid hip hinge and deadlift.

The journey to a barbell deadlift begins in this program with body-weight hip hinges in Phase 1, which will help build mobility and lay the groundwork for good deadlift form. These are followed by dumbbell Romanian deadlifts, which are very similar to hip hinges but add in weight. Finally, we move to the conventional barbell deadlift, which adds bending your knees to get all the way into position to move the weight from the floor.

The barbell deadlift is a real whole-body movement, and it will feel like a lot of things to "think" about at once in terms of positioning all your body parts. But because the whole goal of this program is "teaching your body to move as a functional unit," the barbell deadlift is possibly the most important movement to learn. It is the *ne plus ultra* of lifting weights. Pulling movements are extremely good for your body mechanics, often called upon in real life but difficult to replicate as a training movement without weights. Each opportunity to practice deadlifting is precious.

Deadlift/RDL/hip hinge cues to keep in mind:
- Knees soft, not bending but not locked (for the hip hinge/RDL)
- Feet hip width apart, toes forward or slightly out
- Push hips back like you are trying to close a door with your butt
- Back straight and flat, side to side as well as top to bottom (don't let hips collapse toward the floor; draw them back like a bow)

- Chin tucked, gaze out a few feet in front of you
- Shoulders tucked like you are trying to hold something in your armpits, or prevent someone from tickling you
- No pulling with your arms; they stay straight
- Weight moves in a straight line, not out and around your knees or drifting away from your body

OVERHEAD PRESS

My top real-life reference for overhead press is "putting a suitcase in the overhead bin." But it applies to putting anything on a high shelf, or holding anything up over your head. It's an awkward motion that is hard to do, let alone feel stable while you do it, because your body is so extended. Like the squat, the overhead press is a peak "secret core stability builder."

Overhead presses in weight lifting are less loosey-goosey and more technical than in real life: You hold a weight in your hands in front of you, under your face or chin, and then press it upward using your shoulders and lats. We think of this kind of movement as engaging only our arms, but it's really about the whole shoulder, and to an extent the back, as well as stabilizing the rest of the body

Overhead press is one of the lifts that changes the least throughout the program. For almost everyone, overhead presses are the lift where it becomes difficult to add weight first (because it uses smaller muscles than every other lift). So if that happens to you, don't stress, and refer to the "What to do if you stall" section.

Overhead press cues to keep in mind:

- Feet hip width apart toes pointed forward, weight in your midfoot

- Weight stacked over your forearms
- Chest up, elbows in front of the bar and pointed forward, bar between collarbone and chin, core tight
- The bar should move as close to your face as possible, and your face comes through the "window" of your arms as your extend the weight above your head

ROWS

Bent-over rows are a close relative to the deadlift, in that they are a "pulling" motion, all about bringing stuff closer to your body: opening (or closing) a door, pulling something heavy off a shelf, or, to extend the suitcase metaphor, pulling it off of the conveyor belt after it goes through the security X-ray machine.

Rows are pretty simple: You are holding something out in front of you or below you, and then pulling it toward you using your arms and upper back. Rows come in all shapes and sizes, but in this program we are doing bent-over rows, where we suspend our upper bodies from our bent hips (hip hinge anyone???), let our arms hang down with weights in them, and pull the weights toward our stomachs. There is very little difference between barbell and dumbbell rows.

Row cues to keep in mind:

- Feet shoulder width apart, toes pointed forward or slightly out, knees soft, weight in midfoot
- Hinge at hips like in hip hinge, core tight/engaged, ribs tucked
- Body at 45 degree angle to the floor, grip wider than knees
- With elbows moving at a 30-45 degree angle to your body, pull weight into roughly your belly button,

squeeze shoulder blades together to bring your chest forward, then lower weight back down

OVERHEAD/VERTICAL PULLS (LAT PULLDOWN/PULL-UP WORK)

Vertical pulls, as you may have guessed, are also a "pulling" motion, but they use your muscles in slightly different ways compared to the row. If you've ever wanted to do a pull-up, or pull yourself up from hanging onto a ledge, like Lara Croft, overhead vertical pulls are going to help with that.

This pull involves pulling a weight up or down (depending on whether you are using a machine, or you are the weight, as in a pull-up), using your arms and upper back. Overhead pulls are deceptively difficult; it feels like most people we see doing pull-ups are able to do them with ease, but even for a small to midsized person, a pull-up is effectively lifting, well, your whole body weight. Most people I speak to who are interested in lifting are mostly interested in learning to do a pull-up. This kind of pulling work will get you on the right track, and all of the other lifts here will help to complement it.

Pull-up/pulldown cues to keep in mind:

- The first part of the motion is retracting your shoulder blades (pulling them down and back)
- Aim elbows for your back pocket as well
- Chest up
- Bar comes just below chin
- Control the weight back up until arms/shoulders are fully extended

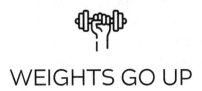

WEIGHTS GO UP

Ahhh, progression. You didn't know it, but this is the thing that virtually every "weight lifting" or "strength building" program you have ever seen is lacking, like the "9-minute strength workout" from the New York Times. They might tell you which moves, how many reps, and how many sets. But without a progression scheme, you are not getting stronger or changing much, really; you are just "working out." Which is fine! But building strength and muscle, whether for the goal of "feeling better in your body" or "changing your body composition," is not possible without a process that absolutely needs a better name, and that process is called "progressive overload."

Progressive overload is a clunky term for predictably increasing the challenge of your training. In the case of this program, we increase the challenge a little bit every single session. This is called "linear progression."

For the purposes of this program we are going to simplify to this core principle: **weights go up.**

"**Weights go up**" means that you add 2.5-5lbs to each lift every session.

But "weights go up" *also* means that you're not jumping into workouts with the aim of running yourself ragged and doing things that are too hard. You are creating the Goldilocks circumstances for sustainable growth, and that means challenging yourself *appropriately*, and taking care to recover from that challenge so you're ready for a slightly bigger challenge next time. Weights can't go up if you start too fast and don't lay a solid foundation in terms of your movement skill.

We do "weights go up"? For three reasons:

1. Too many people seem to think that they are not able to get stronger in any significant way, and it's important for them to know that actually, they can, if they give it a shot!
2. Heavy weights matter. Muscle grows incredibly slowly, and *only if* the weights are appropriately heavy, and you put in the effort to lift them.
3. Mentally speaking, the feedback loop of "weights go up" feels good.

For this reason, once you get to Phases Two and Three, you should strive to add weight to each lift each session.

Add at least 2.5 pounds for upper-body lifts (rows, overhead press, bench).

Add at least 5 pounds for lower-body lifts (squats, deadlifts, RDLs).

If you start out squatting 30 pounds, at your next squat session, you squat 35 pounds. The next time, 40 pounds, and so on. This means even if you start from zero, you will be able to squat a 45-pound barbell after only nine squat sessions.

You might find you CAN add more weight than that, particularly with the lifts that use your bigger muscles, like squats and deadlifts. You might be able to add 10 pounds here and there, or for a while at the beginning, or once you hit a groove. If you are able to do that, or feel like 2.5 pounds is too slow, by all means, go up by 5 or 10 pounds next time. The only thing that really matters is actually pushing yourself on this front, especially if you have long feared heavy weights.

You also might find that the amount you can progress changes as you go. You might be able to jump from the 15 to 25 pound dumbbells early on, only to struggle to go from 60 to 62.5 pounds later. You might also find the reverse; keep in mind that 15 to 25 pounds is a 67 percent jump, while 60 to 62.5 is only 4 percent. If you are struggling with creating reliable progress, check on your form, and see the 'Outside of the gym' section to make sure you are giving yourself the best possible chance at success with your other habits.

As you go from the bodyweight lifts in Phase One to dumbbell-format lifts in Phase Two, and then to barbell format in Phase Three, you may find that your form is a little unsteady, or you can't use exactly the same weights you left off with, because the movements change slightly each time. That is okay and normal; try your lifts with weights you feel confident with first before you continue.

You may also find that at certain points, the next weight jump is too hard. There is no shame in this! In that case, see the "What to do if you stall" section.

KEEP TRACK OF WHAT YOU'RE DOING

You can't change what you don't measure. You might also think, *ehhh, I'll be able to remember what I did last time.* Trust me, you won't. Lifting is a hell of a drug for the brain, and one of the best things about lifting is that it largely prevents thinking in terms of numbers, logic, reason, to-do list items, traumatic memories, and so forth. That means you will not remember next time what you did last time. Go ahead and don't believe me, but you will see. And once you do, just write down what you are lifting so you can refer to it later, and in the longer term, see how far you've come. This is why there is space for numbers and notes in the templates. See the "Recording your workouts" section for more on this.

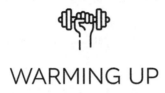

WARMING UP

At this stage of your lifting journey, warming up does not have to be complicated. In Phase One, you don't have to warm up really at all; you can just hop into the workout.

In Phases Two and Three, get your blood flowing for a few minutes before you start by walking on the treadmill or elliptical, doing some light calisthenics (jumping jacks, toe touches, static lunges, whatever moves you). Stretch a bit if you feel tight. This can be a highly personalized process, but some toe touches, lunges, stretching your arms out and back and twisting gently side to side can go a long way, if you haven't moved much yet that day.

In Phase Two, you should begin using "warm-up sets" to work up to your "working weights" for the day for each lift. You might be tempted to skip your warm-up sets in Phases Two and Three, because they feel like extra work; don't! Warm-ups are essential for practicing your form, and can give an early warning that you are feeling off or more tired than usual, allowing you to adjust your working weights if needed.

What do warm-up sets mean? Instead of leaping right into using your 25lb dumbbells for three sets, first you might do a set using the 10s, then a set using the 20s, and then begin your working sets with the 25s.

Isn't this wasting energy? No. It is using more energy that you might have otherwise, but this is all part of the system. Don't skip it. (If you have general anxiety about doing a program with so little cardio, think of this as the cardio you miss so much.)

But okay, those weight amounts seemed random; how are you supposed to know how much weight to use?

In Phase Two, your warm-ups should be like this:

- 5 reps @ 50% of working weight, rounded down
- 3 reps @ 75% of working weight, rounded up
- Begin working sets

So for example, let's say you aim to squat 30 pounds (two 15lb dumbbells) for your 5 sets of 5. To warm up to that point, you would do 5 reps with 15lbs (7.5lb dumbbells), three reps with 25lbs (12.5lb dumbbells), then your working sets.

Especially at smaller weights, these warm-up numbers are not an exact science, so if you don't have weights in increments of 2.5lbs like this, warming up with 10lbs and then 20lbs is fine. Just try to space out two sets before your working weight, and you'll be okay.

You don't need to rest between these sets; the time it takes to fetch the new weights is plenty.

In Phase Three, your warm-ups go like this:

- 5-10 reps with the bare barbell (yes, always start with the bare barbell)
- 5 reps @ 40% of working weight

- 5 reps @ 60% of working weight
- 3 reps @ 80% of working weight
- Begin working sets

If the numbers work out awkwardly and you don't have those plates, round down. Here again, you don't need to rest between these warm-up sets; the time it takes to change the weights is enough rest.

ALWAYS start with the bare barbell in Phase Three. You might feel like no one else in your gym ever does that; that's okay, everyone's on their own journey, however misguidedly macho it may be. You start with the bare barbell.

GENERAL CUES, BREATHING, AND THE SINGULAR JOY OF A REP

Remember: we are looking for good form, not perfect form. All of the cues for the various lifts are a lot to hold in your head all at once, but this is part of developing these movements as skills that you have forever. Eventually, they will become more like reflexes, and you will not have to think quite so much. Ultimately, making time to practice good form is more so the point of this program than banging out rep after rep at any cost. If any of this feels like too much to think about, just do your best to imitate what's happening in the videos, and refer here if your own form looks very off or the movement doesn't feel good.

The love for continuing to study and refine form, the joy in feeling your body move better in new ways, is what keeps bros like myself coming back to lift again and again. "Being good at this already" is not the price of entry. The goal should be to let yourself to take simple, relatively mindless and un-judgmental pleasure in practicing the task itself.

Here are the cues you'll see repeated across many of the different lifts:

During almost all of your lifts, you want your **core tight and "braced."** You do this by **having a small breath held inside you, packed against the spot where your ribs meet (or a couple inches below it)** to create pressure inside of you. Take that breath before you start a rep, hold it there as you move, let it out when you finish the rep, repeat.

To practice bracing, you can lie with your back on the floor, knees bent, resting your hands on your stomach, and practice breathing into your belly slowly. After a few reps of that, practice taking that breath, then gripping it with your core muscles. You can rest a small weight on your stomach to help you see and feel the difference between supporting the weight with a braced core and, for instance, "sucking it in" or just forcing your stomach out hard. This is not something you need to perfect within the scope of LIFTOFF, and it won't make or break your lifting journey by any means. If you continue with lifting, there will be plenty of time to learn and optimize your brace later.

In most cases, the **least-wasteful movement path for any weight will be in a straight line**, as close to the midline of your body as possible. For instance, ideally the barbell in a squat moves in a straight line up and down that is positioned directly over the middle of your foot (just in front of your shoelace ties, probably). In another example, guiding the barbell in an overhead press upward by going way out in front of your face will inherently be more difficult than gliding right by your chin.

"**[Body]weight in your midfoot**" means you're not standing with your weight in your heels, and not in your toes, but in between.

Related to this, many of the videos ask that you "**tuck your shoulders**" in a way that will "rotate the inside of your elbows outward slightly," "**as if you are trying to prevent someone from tickling you.**" This does not mean "pin your upper arms to your sides"; what we are going for is keeping your chest out and engaging your lats. The standing straight arm pulldown motion can help you understand this motion. To do this, stand in front of your good friend, the lat pulldown machine. Set the weight very light—even ten pounds—and grab the bar a few inches outside shoulder width. Keeping your arms straight, pull the bar down until it reaches your body (your upper thighs or crotch region). Control it back up, and repeat for 2 sets of 10 reps.

In lifts that require bringing your chest forward, you will be **retracting your shoulder blades** (like you're trying to pinch something between them). This happens at the top of a row or when you start a deadlift.

For lifts that require creating a shelf with your back to rest your body on, or rest a barbell on, they should be "**retracted and depressed,**" or "**in your back pocket.**" The position you're looking for is the one that comes from **moving your shoulders up, back, and down**; this gives you a solid surface to bench from, and the surface to rest the squat bar on.

Except for arching your back in the bench press (to the extent you're able to; it's not required), strive to **keep your back flat generally**, not just top to bottom but side to side. Don't let your hips collapse toward the floor.

Shoulder/upper back position
(for squatting and benching)

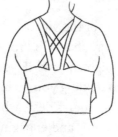

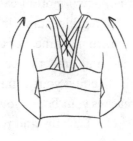

up...

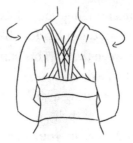

back...

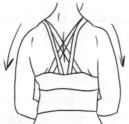

down!

In almost all cases, if you are bending your knees, your **knees should "track over your toes."** This just means they should neither cave way in, nor should you be trying to force them way to the outside of your feet.

Frequently, the instructional videos ask for your **arms/upper elbows to be at a 30-45 degree angle from your body**, or toes to be pointed "slightly out" or "at 30 degrees." These are guidelines, and slightly different angles will be comfortable for everyone; you just don't want your body parts flapping willy-nilly in the breeze.

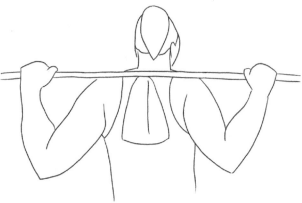

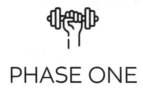

PHASE ONE

Phase One of LIFTOFF has only one type of session that looks like this:

EXERCISE	SETS	REPS
Overhead Press (OHP)	3	8
Bodyweight Squat*	3	10
Incline Pushup**	3	8
Hip Hinge	3	8
Bent Over Row	3	8

LIFTS:

- Bodyweight squat
- Bodyweight hip hinge
- Incline push-up
- No-weight overhead press
- No-weight bent-over row

In addition to the instructions that follow for each of these lifts, you may view instructional videos at couchtobarbell.com/videos.

PROGRESS EVERY SESSION: all progress here is about dialing in your form, so focus on that. Incline push-ups can be incremented by doing them on lower and lower surfaces (a wall, then the back of a chair, then a table, then the seat of a chair, etc.)

REST AFTER EACH SET: 30 seconds, or less if 30 seconds isn't needed

APPROXIMATE TIME PER SESSION: 20 minutes

FREQUENCY: repeat same session 3x/week

YOU WILL NEED:

- A few square feet of space to work out (this workout is easily done at home)
- A broom, Swiffer, length of PVC pipe, or other long, straight, light object
- Surfaces of varying heights, for incline push-ups (a wall, a chair, a table, etc.)

It's true—this first phase of LIFTOFF doesn't even involve any weights, and can be done at home. This phase is specifically designed for people who don't feel quite ready to jump into the potential chaos of a gym right off the bat.

    I didn't generally feel physically awkward in normal life before lifting (well, not more than anyone else). But when I started lifting, I found the way I had to move in the gym fundamentally alien and embarrassing. It felt to me like a lot of sticking my butt and boobs out in pursuit of good form. It took me a while to internalize the idea that what I was doing was normal, nay, strongly encouraged, *inside of a gym*, even if it felt weird generally.

If you are planning on actually entering a weight room at some point, both attuning to an unfamiliar place AND practicing a totally alien, unfamiliar activity can be a lot to handle emotionally at once; it would be like starting a new job you also have no idea how to do. I found that it really, really helped me to separate these things out as much as possible and practice lifts at home to build my confidence, and then add in the task of going the gym.

One of the things that really helped me feel more secure was practicing the movements at home, based on instruction from sources I trusted. This is why Phase One gives you some time to start getting familiar with moving in the ways of weight lifting wherever you're comfortable: your living room, your garage, a bathroom stall in your office; wherever you find time and space.

At this time, we are doing basic versions of our "compound movements" a few reps at a time to start building a foundation of "good form," or using the right muscles all together. You are getting to know the squat, the hip hinge (which will ultimately transform into deadlifts), the push-up (which will ultimately transform into benching), rows, and overhead press. These are the five key movements of lifting weights. Instead of working little individual muscles at once, these compound movements target big muscle groups that are meant to work together day in and out, when you're picking up a box, putting a suitcase into the overhead bin, or nudging furniture around your living room. You are learning to work your muscle groups with the goal of helping yourself move better in your daily life.

Giving your body a little time to learn to move in these ways (at home, with no weights) should only help set you up for success mechanically.

HOW TO START

Before you attempt any workouts, set aside some time to watch through all of the instructional videos linked above and/or in the movement compendium as you start each new phase. If your curiosity is piqued and you want to get up and try the movements as you do this, I'm not going to stop you. But it's important to understand this all as a skill-building process, not just a bunch of workouts, so plan accordingly.

Once you've done that, plan on following along with the videos a bit as you attempt your first workout; that means having a computer or phone on hand. After every set, rest, for 30 or so seconds or until you feel ready. That means you do nothing until you do your next set. Pleasant, isn't it?

It will also help you a lot to try filming your movements to see if you're matching the instructions well enough. You might think you know how to squat or overhead press, but our bodies develop lots of bad habits over years and lifetimes, pressing certain muscles into service while others go dormant (see: bending over and picking things up with our lower backs because our pants are too tight to let us do a proper hip hinge). But that's okay: All the muscles you need are still there, and you can learn!

Some of the movements in Phase One are specifically "barbell"-style movements, but obviously, we are not using a barbell yet. Instead, use any long and light object: a Swiffer, a broom, some PVC pipe, whatever you have lying around. This isn't critical, but being able to hold something in certain cases will help your balance.

This phase of the program is also where you'll learn to "rest" between sets. After each set, you should "rest"; that is, don't do anything except breathe and recover for the next set. This can be as short as 10 seconds or as long as a minute. If you're able to complete each set and need zero rest, it's probably time to move on to the next phase.

The best way to learn to do any of these movements properly will be to do all three sets in a row before starting the next movement.

A MINI-PHASE ONE FAQ

I'm fired up about lifting weights, and I thought this was a weight lifting program, yet I'm looking at the first phase and there are no weights in sight!! Can I skip the first phase if it feels too easy or I'm too excited to start slinging dumbbells around? When am I allowed to go to Phase Two?

You can move on when you are ready to start getting stronger! It's that simple.

I actually, personally believe that a lot more people could start with heavier weights than they think they can. However, many people are just plain scared of weights (if that's not you: Hooray!). Also, most people's form is not that good right out of the gate. You might think you know how to squat, for instance, and think you're ready to leap right into the heavy dumbbells. But you might be wrong, and investing in good form before bringing weights into the picture very much pays off down the line. So do me the courtesy of checking out the movement compendium video first and checking that box before you move on.

I added Phase One specifically because, for me, learning to lift required lots of practice doing the motions without weight anyway, and I might as well have started there. Most resources that have you start with weights will recommend practicing the lifts at home without weight to get the hang of them. This guide is meant to help people starting from zero, and many people might not be starting at actually zero, so we are just building it right into the system.

Phase One also gives you a bit of a time buffer to figure out logistical elements of the rest of the program that you might not have sorted out at the precise moment you arrive here, including "making time to work out." The low stakes of Phase One mean you can jump right in and start practicing lifts now while you find a good gym to join, figure out what a high-protein food and diet look like; how to fit exercising into your schedule; that kind of stuff. That is stuff that does matter and is important to making this whole thing work! By the time you're ready to start making Weights Go Up in Phase Two in earnest, you'll have built up a lot of confidence around the basics, and you'll have streamlined other elements of the whole picture of the learning-to-lift lifestyle.

You might be more mobile or skilled than someone who has never done any strength training before. If you feel like you "get it" and are ready to try you hand at dumbbells, by all means, go for it! Even if you wanted to go right to the barbell movements of Phase Three, be absolutely my guest on that. But this is a program that values skills and form over running you around in circles in order to generate sweat and "burn calories." So if you share those values, invest in them.

I don't care if you can do a shitty squat with crazy-heavy dumbbells; I care that you can do a very beautiful squat with slightly lighter dumbbells that helps you learn to bend down in real life without hurting your lower back.

Whatever you do, remember that getting your form right is key, and that's the main point of Phase One. Your movements don't have to be perfect, and you can continue to work on your form as you learn to use dumbbells, and you can also continue to practice the bodyweight versions of the lifts concurrently with starting to use dumbbells. But if your squat feels like a lot of stress on your knees, or feel your hip hinges mostly in your lower back instead of your hips and hamstrings, proceed with some caution and pay attention to how you're moving; don't get focused on moving weights up at the expense of your form, because it will catch up with you.

I could not disagree more with the question-asker above; Phase One feels too difficult and overwhelming for me right from the get-go. Is there a way to ease in?

First of all, I want to make sure you're not overreaching what is medically safe for you. If Phase One already feels like a lot, please check in with a doctor or your favorite medical professional and make sure you're ready for, as I would describe Phase One to them, some basic bodyweight calisthenics.

If it still just feels overwhelming emotionally, try starting the first week with one set of each movement at a time, and then try going up to two sets in the second week, then three sets in the third. If you are comfortable then, you can move on to Phase Two. If not, repeat that last Phase One week until you are. However, remember that recovery matters here, and if your recovery is right on, no workout should be making you grossly sore or uncomfortable (and even if Phase One workouts feel like a bit much, note that Phase Two drops down to only three movements per day instead of five, with fewer reps per set in most instances).

So it turns out my form is way off on [insert movement]; reviewing my video of myself, it doesn't look right at all and I don't know what to do to fix it! Am I just not cut out for this?

You are cut out for this! Or at least, "struggling with movements you've never done before" is not sufficient evidence that you're not cut out for this. There are two magical things about lifting and building strength and muscle. One, your body *is* naturally built for it; this is basic stuff for your muscles and joints, even if it doesn't feel like it right now. Squats, presses, deadlifts, and the like are the way they are because your body is good at doing them.

Two, being naturally built for it means that your body is always going to be ready to learn again. Your problems are probably attributable to the fact that your body has built up decades of what I will call "range-of-motion debt." That means all you really need is deliberate, consistent practice, versus some sort of special bespoke solution. Sometimes the answer is to be patient with yourself and accept where you are on the lifting journey, today, knowing you are building toward tomorrow. That's all.

While a trainer will be able to tell you specifically, exactly what's wrong, there is often a ton of low-hanging form fruit for someone who is totally new to this. There is very likely nothing wrong with you; don't underestimate how mundane or normal your problems are! You are not alone.

These issues can feel crazy and weird, but it's only because you are generally unfamiliar with the lifting landscape. I've seen a lot the kinds of problems people run into at this stage, and very few are even a little bit unusual. Mostly, they are the same three to five ones for each of the lifts. Mostly, the answer is "keep practicing and you will get there."

If you're struggling with range of motion (that is, no matter what you do, you can't get your body all the way into the right position), log on to your nearest internet portal and search "[movement in question] mobility," which should help you find resources on relevant stretches, and try practicing those along with your workouts. Like strength, you can build mobility and flexibility over time, and you don't need to be God's gift to bendiness to be able to do these movements.

No-weight/barbell overhead press

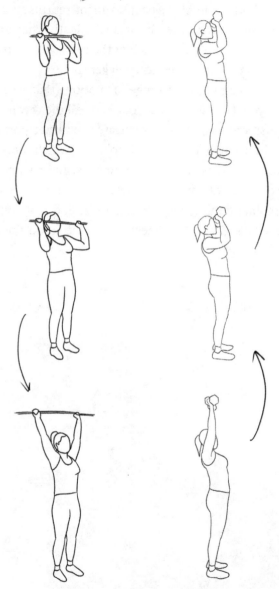

NO-WEIGHT OVERHEAD PRESS

1. Stand with your feet hip width apart, with your weight in the middle of your foot.
2. Hold the bar just outside shoulder width, with the weight resting on your lower palm stacked over your forearms.
3. Lift your chest up, keep your core tight, hips tucked. Elbows should be in front of the bar and pointed forward, with your armpits closed, such that if someone tried to tickle you, they would have a hard time.
4. Take a breath and press it with your core against the inside of your chest right where your ribs meet, keep it there for the rep.
5. Lift the bar as close to your face as possible and bring your face through the window of your arms so the barbell ends above your head.

> Overhead press is a lift where might feel like you can do it "better" however your are used to maneuvering weight over your head. But this way, you learn to use your lats and front delts in a way that is stable and healthy for your shoulders, as well as to keep your body stable when holding something over your head (so no sitting down when you do this movement, either).

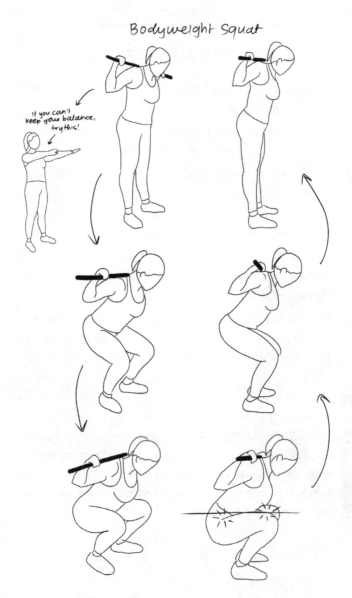

BODYWEIGHT SQUAT

1. You can hold a straight object across your shoulders for balance, but if that feels awkward, you can hold your arms out straight in front for balance, instead.

2. To do a bodyweight squat, and with your heels shoulder width apart; heels will stay on the ground the whole time. Point your toes out 30 degrees, and keep your body weight in your midfoot, chest up, ribs down, and core tight. (These sound like opposing cues, but it just means don't let your chest collapse and hang forward, but neither should you be stretching your core/torso out to max length.)
3. Take a breath and press it against the inside of your chest right where your ribs meet, and keep your core tight.
4. In a controlled motion, sit back in hips as you break at the knees, lower down until hip crease is below the very top of your knees.
5. It's okay if your knees go past your toes, but you want your knees to track over toes, not way inside or outside.
6. Push through the floor and squeeze your hips to come back up
7. in this video I'm pausing at the bottom of the squat. It's okay to move slowly and break down this motion, but work toward instantly reversing the motion as soon as your hip crease gets below the top of your knees.

> If you feel like you're falling backward or forward as your get lower in the squat, to the point that you can't reach full depth—this is a very common issue! Practice squatting while you holding an upright like the side of a door, a door frame, a stair banister or a box right in front of you. Practice resting at the lowest level you can with good form, back flat and straight and heels on the floor, to help teach your muscles to work together, stretch them, and build your depth. As you build your depth, practice releasing your grip on the support in front of you more and more, until you are able to rest in the bottom of your squat with no support.

Incline pushup

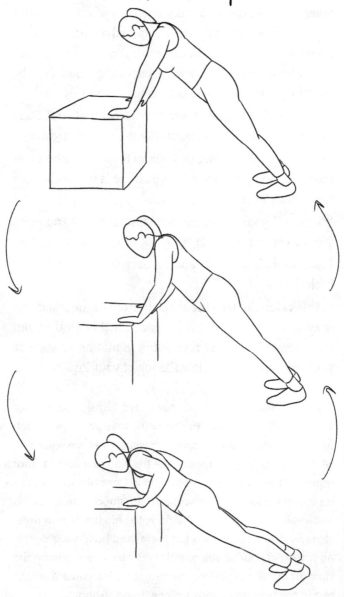

INCLINE PUSH-UP

1. Set up on your toes with your feet hip width apart, hands on the edge of surface or a wall that is a difficult but not all-out effort for your reps. Keep your spine neutral, chin tucked, elbows at a 30-45 degree angle from your body.
2. Take a breath and press it against the inside of your chest right where your ribs meet.
3. With your shoulder blades moving in toward each other together, lower your body down until you are within a fist-width of the surface.
4. Press back up.

> When a set of incline bench reps becomes so easy you could do another set within 30 seconds, progress to a lower surface, until you are doing push-ups right on the floor, if you are able.

Hip hinge

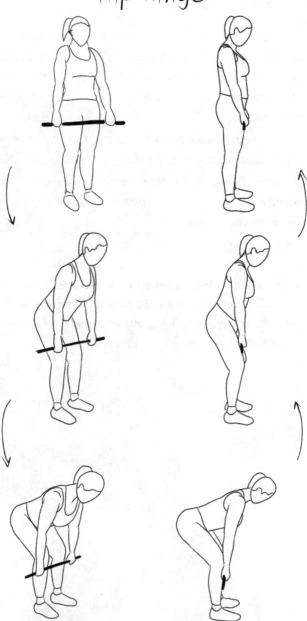

HIP HINGE

1. Stand with your feet hip width apart, knees soft, and your weight in your midfoot. Chest up, ribs tucked down, chin tucked, let your gaze drift with your body as you move.
2. Take a breath and press it against the inside of your chest right where your ribs meet, and hold your core tight.
3. Push back into your hips and fold at the hips like you're trying to close a door or touch a wall with your butt. Push back until you feel a pull in your hamstrings in the back of your legs. Your butt, back, and head should stay flat and in a straight line, you shouldn't be bending at the waist.
4. Squeeze your hip muscles to bring yourself back up. Do NOT pull with your lower back.

> If you struggle with this, stand with your back to a wall and practice touching the wall with your butt by sending your hips back, or hold a stick vertically against your back and make sure your butt, back, and head all stay touching the stick.
>
> The puling feeling in the back of your legs is your cue to stop the motion, but ultimately you want to be able to get your torso parallel to the floor, so go as far as your can at first, and work on increasing the range of motion by holding the position as a stretch for 30 seconds as a cooldown after your workout.

No-weight / barbell row

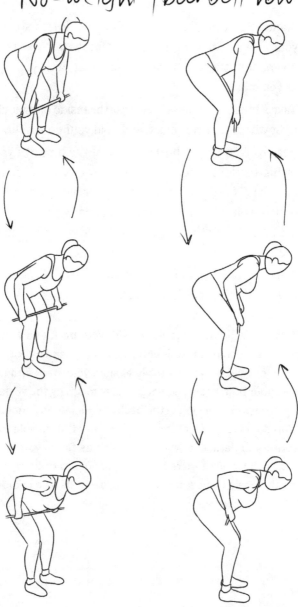

NO-WEIGHT ROW

1. Stand with your feet shoulder width apart, toes pointed forward or slightly out, knees soft, with your body weight in midfoot.
2. Hold the bar with your hands a few inches outside your legs.
3. Hinge at your hips like in the hip hinge, core tight and engaged, back flat, ribs tucked, until your torso is at a 45 degree angle.
4. Take a breath and press it against the inside of your chest right where your ribs meet.
5. With your elbows held at a 30-45 degree angle to your body, pull the weight in toward your body, to about the level of your belly button, and squeeze your shoulder blades together to bring your chest forward.
6. Lower the weight until your arms are fully extended at the bottom.

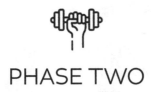

PHASE TWO

Okay here we go: It's weights time, baby.

Phase Two Day A and Day B look like this:

DAY A	SETS	REPS
Dumbbell Squat	5	5
Dumbbell Bench	5	5
Dumbbell Row	3	8

DAY B	SETS	REPS
Dumbbell RDL	5	5
Dumbbell OHP	3	5
Lat Pulldowm	3	8

LIFTS:

- Dumbbell squat
- Dumbbell RDL
- Dumbbell bench press
- Dumbbell overhead press
- Dumbbell bent over row
- Lat pulldown

In addition to the instructions that follow for each of these lifts, you may view instructional videos at couchtobarbell.com/videos.

PROGRESS EVERY SESSION: Add 2.5lbs (upper body) to 5lbs (lower body) to each lift (if you squatted two 15lb dumbbells Monday, squat two 17.5 dumbbells Friday)

REST AFTER EACH SET: 30 seconds-1 minute

APPROXIMATE TIME PER SESSION: 30-40 minutes

FREQUENCY: Alternate two sessions, Day A and Day B, 3x/week (Day A Monday, Day B Wednesday, Day A Friday, Day B Monday, and so on)

YOU WILL NEED:

- A few square feet of space to work out
- Flat shoes to work out in (Converse, Vans, or similar)
- Weights that increment (a full set of dumbbells in 2.5-5lb increments; adjustable dumbbells that go up to at least 25lbs each; or your own DIY weights that you can add a little bit of weight to at a time)

- A lat pulldown machine (or if you don't have that, your long straight object from Phase One + a superband + something overhead to anchor the superband to, such as a door)

Phase Two alternates two different workouts of only three movements each, which is fewer than the five movements of the Phase One workouts. Because of that, Phase Two days may even take less time per day than Phase One. That's why it's all the more important to make sure you are challenging yourself with the weights you use.

Some of the movements from the previous phase will change shape here a little bit, because dumbbells are different than barbells (or in the case of Phase One, fake weightless barbells). Once again, make some time before you get going with this phase to review the Phase Two videos from the movement compendium and do some practice runs in the comfort of your home, especially if it will help with your gym confidence.

An important note here: You do not have to start with the smallest dumbbells possible (in fact, you shouldn't, if you can do more!). Use your first session to experiment with the 10, 15, 20, or even higher-weight dumbbells to find the right starting place for you.

That might look like trying to do squats on Day A with a set of 5lb weights for your first set, finding it too easy, trying a set of 10lb weights, still finding it okay but you're not sure if it's all you can do, and then trying a set of 15lb weights, and finding it too hard. In that case, you can stick with the 10lb weights for next session, and anticipate going up to the 12.5 or 15lb weights the next time you do Day A.

If you aren't in a gym yet and don't have purpose-built equipment, you will have to figure out how to increment your own weights. You can do this with a scale (weigh yourself and the weights) and a little creativity (add books to a backpack that you wear when you squat, for instance). This is going a little off the beaten path and not highly recommended, because I can't account for all the possible movement tweaks that would have to be made here, but use your imagination.

You can simulate a lat pulldown machine with a superband and something to anchor it to overhead, like wedging it in the top of a door. Instead of holding the straps, you can thread your long straight object through the ends and pull down that way. Be careful and stress-test it first. You can also thread something through the band on the other side of the door, like a broom handle, to keep the band from pulling through.

Now that we are integrating weights, tattoo this principle on your heart: **weights go up**. Your goal should be to use a weight that is sufficiently challenging, but not world-ending, for all of the sets you're doing, such that your progress keeps going smoothly. By that I mean: Using weights that are too heavy can lead to bad habits that you will eventually have to fix anyway. You might be able to pick up a 45lb dumbbell and do a squatting motion with it, but you might not hit depth, i.e., get your butt down to the point that your hip crease is below your knees; your knees might cave inward; you might fall a little forward so when you finish the movement you are on your very tippy toes. So be humble and fix your big form issues now (many think lifting weights builds muscle; actually, it builds character).

If I can impart one lesson to you, other than "lifting is good," it would be this: Good form is far more important than raw poundage. No one is impressed by the dudebro unracking 400 pounds and doing a teeny tiny one-eighth-depth squat, except his fellow idiot dudebros.

If you try a weight and it feels way too easy, add 5 or even 10lbs in the next set. But base your progress for the next session on what ended up feeling right.

It might feel tricky to know what feels "too easy" and what feels "challenging," but this is all part of getting to know yourself, and it's good practice for attuning to what is challenging for your body. Try some things out! No one will be hurt by progressing too slowly (though it might frustrate you a little). But keeping the level of difficulty just under "unmanageable" is what will help your body optimally get stronger.

You may also find that, as you go from dumbbell-format lifts in Phase Two to barbell-format in Phase Three, your form is a little unsteady or you can't use exactly the same weights you left off with. That is okay and normal; try your lifts with weights you feel confident with first before you continue the relentless upward trajectory.

If you can't move with some control and confidence, or are feeling the movements in bad or uncomfortable places on your body, the weight is too heavy for you. If that happens:

- Back down the weight to the last weight you could manage
- Revisit the relevant form videos

- Record video of yourself doing the lift to see for yourself (or share with friends who lift)
- If needed, read the "What to do if you stall" section

During this phase, your rest time after each set should get a little longer, as short as 30 seconds and as long as two minutes, but mostly one minute. Technically, you can rest longer, but your workout might start to get bloated with rest time. If you're ready to do your next set a lot sooner than that, up the weights; if you're not even remotely ready after a minute, consider slowing your progression pace.

Try to use two dumbbells of equal weight in each hand, instead of one big one. Sometimes equipment can be scarce, but for the purposes of learning the skill of each movement, keep as many things consistent about the process as possible. This means that, when we talk about progressing your weights, you are adding weight to the total across the two dumbbells, not per dumbbell. So for instance, if you want to start out squatting 20lbs, use two 10lb dumbbells.

When "weights go up" instructs you to add 2.5-5 pounds per lift, you are adding that to the *total* of your two dumbbells, not each dumbbell (though as always, you are always allowed to progress faster if you are able). If you squatted two 10lb dumbbells this session, that is 20 pounds. If you add 5 pounds next session, that would be 25 pounds, or two 12.5lb dumbbells. If your gym doesn't have dumbbells in 2.5lb increments, try first making a bigger jump (10lb dumbbells this session to 15lb dumbbells next session, for instance). You are stronger than you think! If you can't get all your reps with the higher weight, but the lower weight feels too easy, use the rep-based progression scheme in the "What to do if weights won't go up (and a note about OHP)" section.

If you aren't already working out in a gym, now is the time to start scouting out some gym locations in your area, for this reason: A barbell will actually be easier to use than increasingly heavy dumbbells. Beyond a certain point, big dumbbells become unwieldy even for very strong people (ask me and the random 45-pound dumbbell in my house that I sometimes do battle with).

This is also the time to begin eating well in earnest, if you are serious about progressing your weights each session. If your sessions are appropriately challenging, you should be hungry afterward!

WHEN TO GO FROM PHASE TWO TO PHASE THREE

A barbell weighs 45 pounds (20kg), so once you are using the 20-25lb dumbbells for your Phase Two lifts, you are likely ready to move on to Phase Three.

Most of the movements will change slightly going from dumbbells to a barbell, so don't feel discouraged if they feel difficult anew; the barbell is the final weights frontier and will allow you to build strength indefinitely in a way that dumbbells will not. While I'm proud of you for learning to lift 45 or so pounds of dumbbells, you haven't even begun to unlock your potential!

A 70-pound loaded barbell in a bench setup is going to be far, FAR easier for you to handle than two 35-pound dumbbells. This can vary lift to lift; you will be able to hip-hinge much heavier dumbbells than you can squat, overhead press, or bench, for instance. But the good news is, by the time you are reaching the point that you can't maneuver dumbbells anymore, that's probably also right about the time that you will be eminently able to handle a 45lb barbell for the lift in question.

If, at the end of this phase, you are ready to move on to the barbell in some lifts but need to keep using dumbbells for other lifts, that's okay. Keep using the dumbbells for the prescribed reps and sets in Phase Three, and move on to the barbell for the rest. If you are topping out on dumbbells but also struggling with the barbell, try accumulating more reps with the "What to do if you stall" section using the heaviest dumbbells you can currently manage before you make the barbell jump.

I encounter a lot of folks who continue with Phase Two longer than they "should" because they are scared of the gym. That's okay; nothing Bad will happen to you if you keep working with the same weights week after week. But I promised you a whole strength journey, which would not be complete without laying hand to barbell. Barbells, plates, and racks are whole different ballgame, strength-wise. And I seriously want for you not just to keep getting stronger, but to come out of this program feeling comfortable with that set of equipment, ideally in a gym setting. It's normal to balk, but part of the reason we started in Phase One very deliberately at home with low stakes movements was to separate the awkward early learning phases from the gym environment.

Do your best not to be shy about this next phase. Now that you have built up your confidence and laid the lifting knowledge foundation, I hope you feel ready to tackle the weight room in the gym.

Okay, I have no idea how strong I am. Where do I start in terms of weights?

Return to the gospel: "weights go up." **Use as heavy of weights as you can manage, while still maintaining good form, that you are able to recover from and challenge yourself more next time.** This means you can start with whatever feels challenging but not world-ending for you to do for the number of reps dictated by the program. If you attempt a weight for your first set and it feels way too easy, add 5 or 10 pounds to the next set.

The definition of "challenging" within beginner strength training (that is, during linear progression) is "with one or two reps left in the tank during your set," or "RPE 8" (i.e. your "rate of perceived exertion" is an 8 out of 10); that is to say, you could do a little more within the set you're doing, but not lots and lots more. This is a hard line to identify when you are using your body in this new way. The only way you will find it is by experimenting.

If a weight feels heavy but you suspect you can do more than the number of reps you should be doing, try and keep going beyond those reps and see how many you can get. If it's over two times as many reps as you should have done (you're supposed to do 8, but could easily do 16 or more), go up next session or set by at least 5 pounds. If it's over 1.5 times (you're supposed to do 8, but could easily do 12), go up by at least 2.5 pounds.

These aren't hard and fast rules, but a little bravery and experimentation is the only way you're going to find out what you're capable of. Don't be a hero, don't do anything dangerous, and don't sacrifice your good form. But DO open your mind to the possibility of failure as a way of understanding yourself and your journey, without it defining you.

I've been able to do this program through Phase Two at home so far, but now I can't go up in weight any more without starting Phase Three and going to a gym. However, I'm scared. Can I just keep doing Phase Two forever?

Theoretically, you can just keep going with any one of these phases pretty much forever. It's just that at a certain point, you're not being challenged anymore, and the whole endeavor goes from being "progress" to being "exercise and/or maintenance." You won't be getting stronger, you won't be changing the size or capability of your muscles, you'll just be moving for a certain amount of time each week. This makes the path to recomposition or knowing how much to eat less clear, which is fine. But if those parts matter to you, going into a holding pattern means stepping off that track fro a bit.

Maybe that's fine for you! But I will say, I can't promise you will really understand the whole muscle-building trajectory and experience if you don't eventually move through all the levels. If you feel like doing incline push-ups is always hard because you don't eat enough food and protein to build strength, you might never move onto using dumbbells or a barbell. If that never happens, you'll never find out that, with the right amount of steady incremental progress, it doesn't actually feel that much harder to lift 70 pounds, or a hundred pounds, or 135 pounds, than it did at one point to do a single push-up. I'm not kidding, it really is that magical. But you have to give it a chance.

So the answer is, yes you can, but also, I hope you can find your way to the next phase when you feel ready. There is a whole section just for you coming up, titled "How to start going to the gym."

Dumbell squat

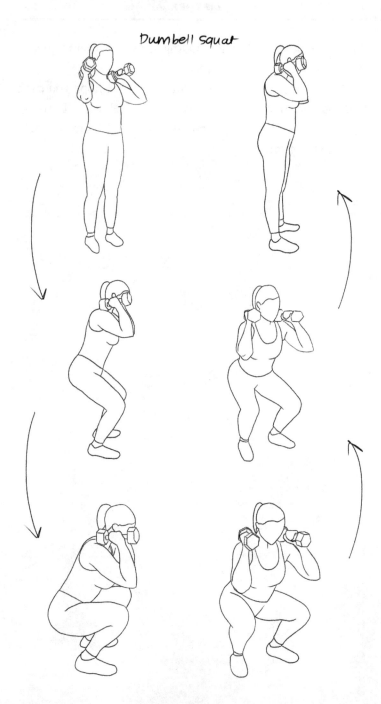

DUMBBELL SQUAT

1. Stand with your heels shoulder width apart; heels will stay on the ground the whole time. Point your toes out 30 degrees, and keep your body weight in your midfoot, chest up, ribs down, and core tight.
2. Hold your dumbbells so one end rests on either shoulder.
3. Take a breath and press it against the inside of your chest right where your ribs meet
4. Sit back in your hips as you break at the knees, lower down until your hip crease is below the very top of your knees
5. It's okay if your knees go past your toes, but your knees should track over your toes, not inside or outside.
6. Push through the floor and squeeze your hips to come back up.

Dumbell bench

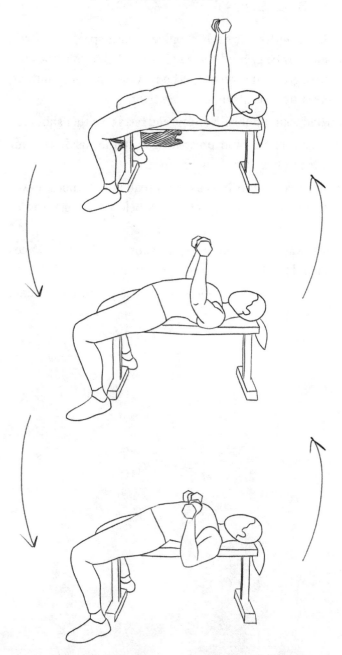

DUMBBELL BENCH

1. While sitting on the bench, hold the dumbbells in your hands standing one dumbbell on end on each leg.
2. Kick each dumbbell up to shoulder height just in front of your face, and roll back to lie down. (This is easier than other ways of trying to lie down and get the weights in the right position; may take some practice, but it's a skill you'll use again and again!)
3. Push the dumbbells up in the air to full extension, and while holding them steady, scooch around to shift your shoulders up, back, and down, so the place your back is resting is toward the tops of your shoulder blades, will create an arch in your back. (You can practice this without weights if needed, and be sure to practice it with your warm-up weights.)
4. With your elbows at a 45 degree angle to your body, lower the dumbbells until the bottom surface of them is even with your chest.
5. Press the weights up and together.
6. When done with your reps, you can roll up with the dumbbells in the same position you used to lie down with them, or just carefully drop them to your sides.

Dumbell row

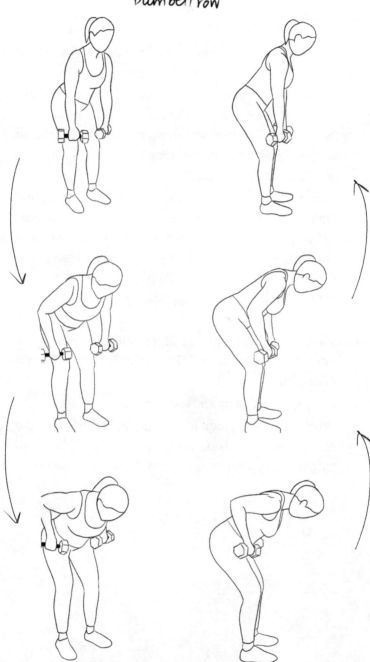

DUMBBELL ROW

1. Stand with your feet shoulder width apart, toes pointed forward or slightly out, knees soft, and your body weight in your midfoot.
2. Hinge at the hips as in the hip hinge and then rest at the bottom of the movement, core tight/engaged, back flat, ribs tucked until you reach a 45 degree angle to the floor.
3. Your arms should hang loose, but rotate your shoulders back like you are turning the inside of your elbows slightly forward, like you are trying to prevent someone from tickling you.
4. Take a breath and press it against the inside of your chest right where your ribs meet
5. With your elbows held at a 30-45 degree angle to your body, pull the dumbbells in toward your body, at about the level of your belly button, and squeeze your shoulder blades together to bring your chest forward.
6. Extend your arms fully back to the bottom of the movement.

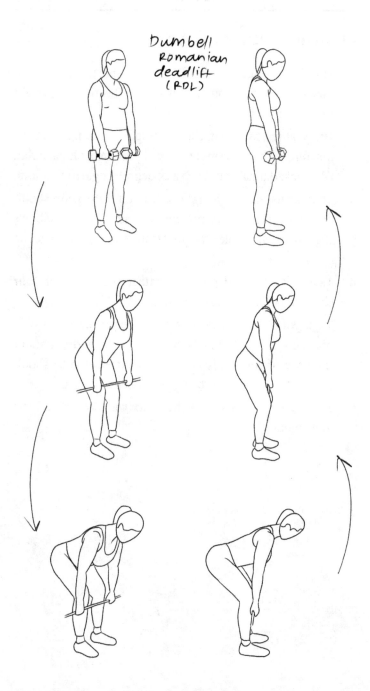

DUMBBELL RDL

1. Stand with your feet hip width apart, knees soft, and your body weight in your midfoot.
2. Take a breath and press it against the inside of your chest right where your ribs meet. Keep your core tight chest up, ribs down, chin tucked, gaze drifting as you move your body.
3. Your arms should hang loose, but rotate your shoulders back to engage them, like you are turning the inside of your elbows slightly forward, like you are trying to prevent someone from tickling you.
4. Push back into your hips as your keep your back flat until you feel a pull in your hamstrings in the back of your legs, or until the dumbbells are just below your knees.
5. Squeeze your hip muscles to bring yourself back up. Do NOT pull with your lower back.

> As with the hip hinge, your butt, back, and head should stay in a straight line, with your torso suspended from your hips, you should **NOT** be bending at the waist. If you don't have the range of motion to get the dumbbells below your knees, go as far as you can with good form until you feel that hamstring stretch in the back of your legs. This will help develop your range of motion.

Dumbell overhead press

DUMBBELL OVERHEAD PRESS

1. Stand with your feet hip width apart, toes pointed forward, your body weight in midfoot. Hold your dumbbells to either side/just in front of your neck, weight resting on your lower palm stacked over your forearms, elbows 45 degrees to your body and in front of the weight, pointed forward with armpits closed such that if someone tried to tickle you, they would have a hard time.
2. lift chest up, ribs down, core tight, hips tucked.
3. Take a breath and press it against the inside of your chest right where your ribs meet.
4. Press weights up until your arms are fully extended over your head, then bring them back down.

Lat pulldown

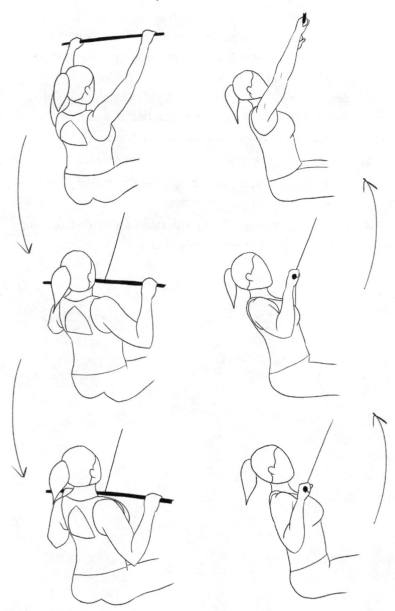

LAT PULLDOWN

1. Grab the bar or handles 6-10 inches outside shoulder width grip.
2. From standing, lower yourself to sitting, bar in your hands.
3. Lean backward slightly so that your chest is pointing up, and keep it pointing up throughout the movement. Resist the temptation to cave it down and inward; this is what keeps this back-and-arm movement from turning into just an arm movement.
4. Retract your shoulder blades as you keep your elbows at 45 degrees, pulling the bar down to between your chin and your upper chest as your pull your elbows "together" toward the sides of your body at the bottom.
5. Control the bar back up to the top.

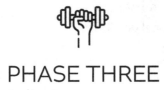

PHASE THREE

Finally, after all your weeks of hard work, it's time to touch barbell.

Phase Three Day A and B look like this:

DAY A	SETS	REPS
Barbell Squat	5	5
Bench	5	5
Bent Over Row	3	8

DAY B	SETS	REPS
Barbell Deadlift	3	5
Overhead Press	3	5
Lat Pulldowm	3	8

LIFTS:

- Barbell high-bar squat
- Conventional deadlift
- Bench press
- Overhead press
- Lat pulldown (or pull-up progression; see Resources and FAQ)
- Bent-over rows

In addition to the instructions that follow for each of these lifts, you may view instructional videos at couchtobarbell.com/videos.

PROGRESS EVERY SESSION: Add 2.5lbs (upper body) to 5lbs (lower body) to each lift (if you squatted 50lbs Monday, squat 55lbs Friday, 60lbs the following Wednesday, and so on)

REST AFTER EACH SET: ~1 minute

APPROXIMATE TIME PER SESSION: 40 minutes

FREQUENCY: alternate two sessions, Day A and Day B, 3x/week (Day A Monday, Day B Wednesday, Day A Friday, Day B Monday, and so on)

In this phase, we will be returning to many of the form videos from Phase One. But instead of our Swiffer, a barbell (45lbs) will be in its place.

For this phase, you will need at minimum:

- Rack(s) for squatting and benching
- A barbell
- Flat sneakers for working out in (Converse, Vans, or similar)
- A set of weight plates that accommodate your strength level
- Room to deadlift
- A lat pulldown setup of some kind

Ideally, you would have these specific versions of the above (and having any of them is better than having none):

- A power or squat rack with adjustable pegs and safety arms, with holes in the uprights that allow to set those pegs and arms at a range of heights
- An Ohio Power Bar or similar, with medium-grade knurling
- Flat sneakers for working out in (Converse, Vans, or similar)
- A set of weight plates that include light bumper plates for use in deadlifting
- A platform for deadlifting (dedicated lifting gyms will have this; Planet Fitness will not)
- Clips for the ends of the barbell, to hold plates in place
- A lat pulldown machine

This phase is probably about the time you will transition to a gym, if you didn't already in the previous phase. I know that, for many of you, this is the scary part. But look at me in my two eyes: You've got this. For tips on that process and what to look for in a gym, see the "When to go to a gym" section.

This phase also introduces full range-of-motion conventional deadlifts, after spending eight weeks practicing our hip hinges and Romanian deadlifts. This is it: the time you learn how to lift with your legs, not your back. If you struggle with conventional deadlifts, particularly setup and equipment, see the "A note on deadlifts" section. If you struggle with overhead press, and/or your gym only has weights in 5lb or greater increments but you need smaller increments to progress, see the "What to do if weights won't go up (and a note about OHP)" section. If you struggle with squat depth, see the "A note on squat depth" section.

Rows, overhead presses, and the lat pulldown are essentially the same as in prior phases. No additional instructions are required; refer to previous sections to revisit them if you need.

Rests in this phase should be about the same as they were in Phase Two. One minute is a good sweet spot. If you're ready to do your next set a lot sooner than that, up the weights; if you're not even remotely ready after a minute, consider slowing your progression pace or checking in on your recovery (see the "Outside of the gym" section for this).

Once you've completed this phase: Congrats, you are now a barbell-literate member of swole society! You will walk in and out of the weights section of the gym with ease; racks of plates will part like the Red Sea as you approach; your limbs are at your command. When this phase is over, if you want guidance on what to do next, refer to the "What's next" section.

Barbell squat

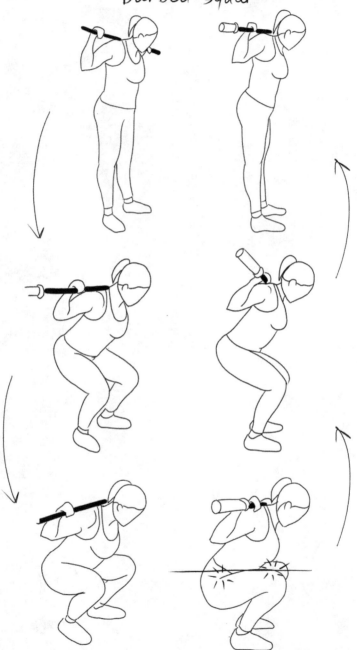

BARBELL SQUAT

1. Set up the rack and hooks so they are holding the barbell at about level with your armpits.
2. Face the barbell, and grip it about 6 inches outside shoulder width grip on either side.
3. While holding onto the barbell, bring your upper body under and around to the other side of it, and move your shoulders up, back, and down to set your upper back in a tight position, as in the dumbbell or barbell bench. Press the barbell into the tops of your. The barbell should be pressed into your trap muscles at the base of your neck, and supported by, but not grinding into, your shoulder bones.
4. Use a small squat motion to get the weight up and out of rack using your legs and take 3 steps back--one foot back, other foot back, first foot back to be even with second foot.
5. Your heels should be shoulder width apart and stay on the ground, toes pointed out 30 degrees.
6. Stack the weight of the barbell over your midfoot, and shift your weight to be in your midfoot, chest up, ribs down.
7. Take a breath and press it against the inside of your chest right where your ribs meet and keep your core tight.
8. Sit back in your hips as you break at the knees, lower down until hip crease is below the very top of your knees.
9. Track your knees over your toes; it's okay if your knees go past your toes.

10. As you go down and come back up, the barbell should move in a straight line over your midfoot.
11. Press into the floor and squeeze your hips to bring yourself back up.
12. When you're done, walk the barbell back into the rack until your feet are together and the barbell meets the uprights, then drop it to the pegs by squatting it down.

> When you transition from the dumbbell squat to the barbell squat, the weight is positioned quite differently relative to your body—the dumbbell squat has the weight more forward, while the barbell squat rests the weight on your back. This will take some adjustment, but that is very normal, so don't be discouraged! It may help to go back to practicing squatting with a broom or other sticklike object. You should also make sure to do your warmup sets, and use a rack with safety arms if you feel unsteady with the barbell.

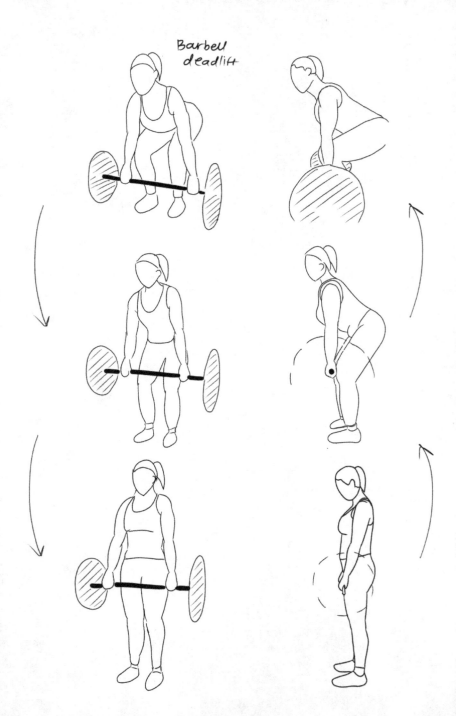

BARBELL DEADLIFT

1. Stand in front of the barbell loaded on the ground. If you are deadlifting less than 135 pounds, the bar should still be at the same height it would be with 45 pound plates on each side (about mid-shin, for most people). If your gym does not have bumper plates that are lighter but the same size as standard 45lb plates, use risers or other equal surfaces to boost the barbell's height up.
2. Stand with your feet hip width apart, toes straight or slightly pointed out, bar stacked over midfoot (just in front of your shoe lace ties), with your weight in midfoot.
3. Without moving the barbell, you are going to bending yourself around it as you pull yourself toward it. Push your hips back as in your hip hinge, and reach down to grab the barbell at shoulder width just outside of your knees.
4. Bend your knees and hips and bring your chest through your shoulders until your shins meet the unmoving barbell. Rotate your shoulders back like you are turning the inside of your elbows slightly forward and closing your armpits, like you are trying to prevent someone from tickling you.
5. From the side view, your shoulders will be in front of the barbell, and your shoulder blades will be directly over the barbell; if this isn't the case, adjust until it is.
6. Tuck your chin and gaze out a few feet in front of you.
7. Take a breath and press it against the inside of your chest right where your ribs meet. You will hold this breath there for the whole rep.

8. As you pull yourself into position, you should hear the barbell tense and click against the plates. This is the "slack" being pulled out of the barbell.
9. Check that your core is braced, chest up, ribs down, arms straight, back flat and straight (both top to bottom as well as side to side; don't let your hips droop or cave toward the floor).
10. Stand up with the weight in your hands, with the barbell keeping contact with your legs the whole way. You are NOT pulling with your lower back, but keeping tension in your back and hips while extending your knees and hips at the same time, driving the floor away from you. The barbell should move in a straight line against your legs, with your knees extending to move out of the way of that straight line. Continue to extend until your are standing straight with the barbell in your hands.
11. Once you get to the top, break at the hips and hold onto the barbell as you release it to gravity and control it down to the floor.

Barbell bench

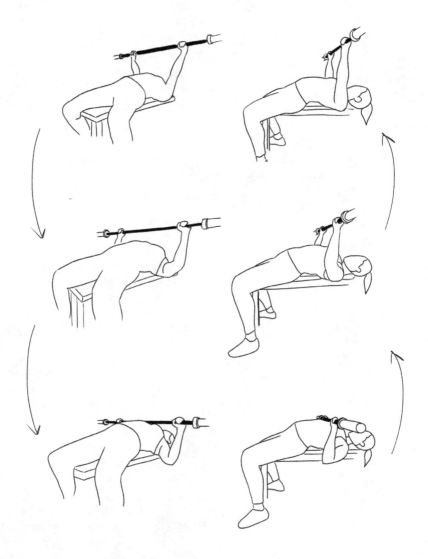

BARBELL BENCH

1. Lie back on the bench so the bar is roughly aligned with your eyes.
2. Move your shoulders up, back. and down so the place your back is resting on the bench is toward the tops of your shoulder blades. This will help create a small arch in your back.
3. Grab the barbell 6-10 inches on each side outside shoulder width grip, so the bar is in your mid-to-lower palm, and then wrap your fingers around it.
4. Press barbell up out of pegs and bring it out so it is stacked over your shoulders and the bar is stacked over forearms so that it's not bending your wrist back.
5. In a controlled motion, keeping your elbows at a 45 degree angle to your body, lower the bar to the bottom of your pecs, or about where the bottom band of your bra sits.
6. Rest the barbell there for a moment, and then, keeping your elbows at that angle, press it back up. Don't shift your shoulders out of position. The barbell should move roughly in a straight line, or a line that slants slightly backward to the rack.
7. Repeat for all your reps, then rack the bar by moving it straight back toward the uprights first, and then dropping it into the hooks.

WHEN TO GO TO A GYM

SO WHEN DO I ACTUALLY GO TO A GYM? DO I EVEN NEED A GYM?

Phase One of this program is easily doable without a gym, as long as you have space and some sort of stick to practice with.

Phase Two gets trickier, but if you have at-home weights or can fashion makeshift weights from stuff you have at home that you can also increment (e.g., you can add a 5lb book to a backpack you hold or wear while you do squats), you can get away without a gym there as well.

The last phase will be the hardest to accomplish without a gym. You can buy your own weights, but barbells and plates are unfortunately fairly expensive. So unless you happen across a fire sale at a gym that's going out of business, you will probably have to find somewhere to go in order to complete the program. Therefore, if you are just starting this program, plan on seeking out a gym between three and eight weeks from now, depending on whether you have or can get weights at home.

The good news is that there is probably a gym better suited to this program than you think, closer than you think, and cheaper than you think. Strength-training-focused gyms are usually less slick than and don't advertise as well as your local globo-gym, but they can be equally welcoming, as well as inexpensive! For the first three years I lifted, I paid $15 per month to Richie's Gym, a shabby black iron haunt in Bushwick beloved by locals, especially the firefighters who worked at the firehouse around the block. When I needed to visit my hometown of Albany but wanted to keep training, I was pleasantly surprised to learn that for years there had been a gym perfect for strength training in the area, called Albany Strength, that charged all of $5 for a day pass and required no contracts. I wouldn't have known it was there because I didn't know what to look for; once I did, it appeared.

One option that will be a relatively sure bet to get access to the right equipment is current or former CrossFit gyms. They might have limited hours, but they are run fairly independently and have something called "open gym hours" when they aren't doing classes and anyone can use the equipment. If you explain you are just looking to train on your own, the owner might cut you a membership deal (CrossFits are painfully expensive normally, I know). Failing that, try asking around. If you see a gym bro around your bougie globo-gym, ask her where she works out.

SIGNS THAT A GYM ISN'T SUITED TO LIFTING HEAVY WEIGHTS

Any bans on grunting or banging weights. Weights are loud; anyone who respects training knows this. It's not reasonable to expect people not to make a little noise.

Only Smith machines, no free-weight racks. You've probably seen these before, most likely at your globo-gym. They look like they let you learn to do squats or bench without any of the scary parts, like balancing the weight with your body. Unfortunately, that is a crucial element of what makes strength training good in the first place. Free weights matter. It's none of my business if a gym wants to have a Smith machine, but the gym should also have racks, ideally power racks with adjustable pegs and safety arms for any height, a freely moving barbell, and plates to load onto that barbell. See the "Terms" section for more on what these things are.

Fixed-height pegs on the bench/squat racks. This isn't the worst thing in the world; Richie's had only fixed-height pegs on its squat and bench racks, and I made it work. But basically, you are trying to minimize how much you have to maneuver barbells when unracking them at the start of a set. If the pegs are extremely low and you basically have to do half a bench or squat rep to get them out of the rack, that's not ideal (and you *never* want to have to hyperextend or stand on your tiptoes to unrack a weight). A power rack should have incremental holes all the way up and down its uprights so you can adjust the pegs and safeties to the right height for you.

Lack of bumper plates. This is another one that's not strictly a dealbreaker, but a gym with bumper plates (plates that are the same size as regular 45lb plates, but lighter) will make it much easier to learn to deadlift. You are much more likely to find these at a sport-specific gym or current/former CrossFit box. Please see "a note about deadlifts" if you don't have access to bumper plates.

HOW TO GO TO THE GYM, EMOTIONALLY SPEAKING

Read this every time before you go, if you need:

You pay the same gym membership fee as everyone else.

You are here for a normal and good purpose, to have a fun time, to challenge yourself and build your skills, and that is what gyms are for. Presumably you want to get strong as hell, and that is also what gyms are for.

We all went to kindergarten and have a reasonable expectation that each other knows how to share and take turns.

Most people who lift weights, just like most people in general, are probably nice and normal people who are not really thinking about you or what you are doing, even if they seem to be staring in your direction. I have done this many times, but all I'm doing is resting and spacing out, or thinking about my next set.

Here are some behaviors of other gym patrons that are their problem, not yours: monopolizing equipment; freely commenting on your form; unsolicited spotting; anything that makes you feel uncomfortable. These things do suck, but they are not unique to the gym, and you are entitled to dislike them and report them to gym staff.

If someone tries to make unsolicited commentary or have a conversation you're not interested in, you are allowed to pretend you are on an important phone call taking place in your headphones and can't hear them. Not now. You have Milan on the line.

If you don't have headphones, you are allowed to nod and smile and say "OK!" noncommittally throughout the interaction and then just go back to what you were doing.

Everyone in the gym didn't know what they were doing at some point. You are allowed to learn and grow and fuck things up just like everyone else.

You might feel like you don't even know where the right place to stand is without getting in other people's way. It's okay; you will learn. Learning to do this basic thing is well within your grasp, but "never making a mistake" is impossible.

You are allowed to make noise. You are allowed to stick your butt and boobs out if proper form demands it (or whenever else you feel like it). You are allowed to sweat and grunt and strain. You are allowed to fail. You are human. These are things humans do, and the whole point of gyms is to give humans a place in which to do them.

I'M STRAIGHT UP SCARED OF THE WEIGHT ROOM AND I FEEL LIKE THAT WILL NEVER, EVER CHANGE. WHAT DO I DO?

I hear you. This was a far bigger obstacle for me to overcome than a lot of other hangups I had about lifting. Weight rooms can feel like unfamiliar territory that belongs to someone else.

But I have to tell you, while your feeling is valid, it will not serve you in this journey. The weight room belongs to you, too, and you cannot let assholes who disagree (the few of them that there are!) have the upper hand and control your life.

First—don't assume everyone in there is an asshole. I thought everyone would be an asshole at Richie's Gym, and then practically no one was an asshole. I was surprised how much I was left alone, and how many actually positive interactions I had. Give them a chance; they may not be so bad!

Sure, there will be the occasional asshole in there, but there are assholes everywhere. In New York I practically bump into an asshole every day before I'm even all the way out of the door to my apartment. I know it feels like a particular injustice to have to endure assholes WHILE you do something that feels as vulnerable as "trying to learn to lift weights," but as in the rest of your life, I hope you aren't letting assholes scare you away from some of the best parts of living. You shouldn't have to bear this responsibility, but, consider reporting assholes to the gym staff. Assholes: Stop being assholes. Everyone else: You have a reasonable expectation of people not being assholes.

Second, everyone started somewhere, even the assholes. And while those assholes probably benefited from having a big daddy asshole who took them under their wing and showed them the weight room ropes, they're still all assholes. You don't have to be, and you can play a part in making that room no longer assholes-only.

I NEVER FEEL READY TO GO UP IN WEIGHT, AND/OR I TRIED IT AND VERY EMBARRASSINGLY FAILED A REP AND DROPPED THE DUMBBELLS/BARBELL IN FRONT OF EVERYONE, MAKING VERY LOUD NOISES! I AM PISSED, I AM STRESSED, I HATE MYSELF, I WANT TO GIVE UP! IT MIGHT BE BECAUSE THE JUMP FROM ONE WEIGHT TO THE NEXT FEELS TOO BIG, AND MY GYM DOESN'T HAVE SMALLER WEIGHTS.

I get it; this is very frustrating! But here is the thing: Life has setbacks, and so does lifting. All we can do is troubleshoot, have patience, and keep trying. This is all part of the process; I swear it to you on my own set of plates. You are surely not the first person to get stuck, and you won't be the last. Refer to the "What to do if you stall" section for how to get unstuck.

And don't be embarrassed, because this is what lifting IS. Lifting means trying, failing, and experimenting. This is exactly why I love it; I can't stand doing complex and frenetic high-step kick-ball-change moves where I'm desperately trying to keep up with an instructor. I love to monastically study the universe-in-a-grain-of-sand that is a body trying to do a mechanically sound squat.

While I've leaned pretty hard on the "Weights go up" argument elsewhere in this book, progress is *also* gaining awareness and skill with the way that you move, making it better and more sound each time. You might actually have been born a decent squatter, but now your body has been run through years of tight pants, a sedentary job, and overall embarrassment about the prospect of ever sticking your butt out too much. Getting back in touch with the way your body wants to move, the way it moves well, is extremely valuable and worthwhile work, and that's what you're doing when you learn to lift heavy weights.

Once you're using a barbell, other than the "stall" protocol in the "What to do if you stall" section, one option is buying fractional plates of your own, in 2.5lbs or 1.25lbs sizes. A pair of the latter is pretty light and cheap, and you can keep them in your gym bag. Having two pairs of those plates of your own will allow you to work in increments of 2.5lbs.

If you try this and are still failing anyway, your recovery may be the issue. You must eat, you must drink water, and you must sleep. If you are failing but think you are eating enough, you are probably wrong. Eat more. Add an extra snack. Have some toast and nut butter before the gym. Have a protein shake before bed. Have lunch dessert. Pick one of these things and see if it helps.

HOW TO START GOING TO THE GYM

At various other points in this book, I have encouraged/warned you that it'll be hard to complete this program without going to a gym eventually. Some people are able to keep Phase Two at home by investing in some adjustable dumbbells (I'd recommend getting a set that goes up to at least 25 pounds per hand, if you do). But it's not reasonable to expect most people to get a full barbell/rack/plates setup in their house; that's very expensive, and it's not unheard of for such objects to put holes in your walls/floors/ceiling. No judgment on when you choose to hop into the gym environment.

To that end, for whenever it happens here are some comprehensive instructions on getting situated with a new gym. It takes pains with the details, because I know what it's like to be terrified/mortified/paralyzed by a new, unfamiliar environment.

But the important thing to remember, as I will stress throughout, is that the gym really is a new place like any other: a new school, a new workplace, hell, even a new grocery store. Where is the milk? Where are the produce bags? How do I print something? Why is the door to the place I have to go locked? Is the pool really on the roof? And so forth. As in all those situations, you will have to take some deep breaths, find in yourself some patience, and remember that this is not a problem with you; you are *going to figure it out*, I promise. And with each subsequent session, you'll get more and more comfortable.

HOW TO START GOING TO THE GYM, PART 1: THE CASE FOR THE GYM VISIT

While gyms have some similarities with other places, I admit: they can be intimidating. They are unfamiliar; they can be chaotic; they have myriad unwritten rules, such as "Stand ONLY here to do deadlifts, and NEVER stand here to do dumbbell curls, lest you be in foot traffic." There are invariably some people making noises that sound like two silverback gorillas fighting. This all costs money, somehow. All these unique elements make gyms ecosystems for which neither school, nor family, nor even gym class adequately prepares us.

I am someone who is inherently initially uncomfortable in any new environment. Spiritually, and sometimes literally, I have to pin myself to the wall and observe the habitat, in order to be sure I am rewarding none of my enemies with the element of surprise. Only after a nice chunk of time spent watching do I feel barely assured enough that there are no imminent threats.

Even some of the most confident and self-assured people I know are like, "Gyms? No thank you. I will work out ONLY in a private stall, obscured from view."

The situation of "starting to go to the gym" is a rare instance where I feel everyone may benefit from behaving as awkwardly as I do generally, trying to disappear into the wall as you watch. By that I mean: you should separate out the mental task of "going to a new place" from all the other hurdles that getting started with working out involves.

We often think of "starting to work out" as just one, fairly easy, task. But it's actually three incredibly annoying tasks:

1. Going to a new place
2. Sorting out the logistics of your workout in a new place (including schedules/timing)
3. Putting the pieces together and actually doing your own entirely new workout

That's too many tasks at once. I say do one at a time.

It may seem like a weird time to publish this, when very few people are going to the gym. But that's just the thing: the BEST time to ease yourself into gym-going is when not many other people are gym-going. The dead of summer, the dead of winter (though crucially, NOT January)—these are the times when you will feel a little more room to breathe.

Therefore, let's start with the first step: availing yourself of what I'm going to call a "gym visit."

HOW TO PULL OFF THE GYM VISIT

Firstly, you must go to the gym with no expectation of really accomplishing anything. You are just going in order to take in the atmosphere, to people-watch, to vibe-assess.

That doesn't mean you go and appear to do nothing, standing there slack-jawed in the middle of the room staring unblinkingly at the guy on the AbCoaster (so named because it is more like a carnival ride than a workout). Obviously, you *pretend* to work out. You do *nominal motions* of working out. To the untrained, glancing eye, you *are* working out. But in reality, you are just doing recon. This visit is almost strictly anthropological in nature.

Pursuant to that: secondly, you must watch. Are you curious where people usually squat, or how they adjust the racks? Where they stand to do dumbbell work? Where is the cleaning stuff? What does it look like when someone is resting between sets? How do people "work in" with one another? DOES anyone actually get hectored by any of the bros, or are the bros in fact nice, peaceable, even supportive guardians of the workout machine forest? If you give yourself 20 or 30 minutes of observation time, you can learn all these things.

If the treadmills are too out of the way, try to quickly identify some of the least-used machines to sit on. Ab crunch machines, lat raise machines, and pec flye machines tend to be very little-used; chest press machines are used sometimes, but there tend to be way too many of them. All of these are effectively fancy chairs. Set them to the lowest possible weight and pretend to do reps, and "rest" between sets while you observe. Identify a new underused machine and move after several minutes. No one will be the wiser or care that your workout seems to consist only of ab crunches, lat raises, and pec flyes.

How to make sure you are assessing a gym's true chaos? Go when you'd go normally in your routine, if you know when that is. If you don't, try to go at a reasonably busy time, which will usually be "after-work-ish until an hour or two before closing," like 4-8 p.m. In an empty gym at 5 a.m., there will be nothing to observe. The empty gym is actually best for the next step, when you start sorting out the logistics of your workout.) If you are not typically free during this time, it doesn't matter; you only really need to do this once, though you can technically do it as many times as it takes you to feel comfortable. Also, in the low seasons, the gym is always going to be less chaotic than on, say, January 2, but if you start now, you'll be prepared for the chaos by then.

But how to get the gym to let you do this? Most gyms, even the dreaded Planet Fitness, will let you visit once, or get a three-day pass, or pay for a day pass, without signing up for a membership. This is the perfect way to do a vibe check on the gym.

This is also the perfect way to procrastinate actually starting your workout regimen, and I know at least a few people are into that.

So that's it! That's all of step one. Next week we'll do step two (layering in logistics), and after that, if you can believe it, step three (actually accomplishing your workout).

HOW TO START GOING TO THE GYM, PART 2: THE PRE-PRODUCTION DRY RUN

At this point, you've visited, you've gotten the lay of the land, you've perhaps even reassured yourself that the gym not a competitive conflict-heavy hellscape ruled by bros blind with PED-fueled rage, but a bunch of people mostly minding their own business. So now it's time to dip a toe into the gym waters and actually attempt the motions of your workout.

It might seem like this should be the second of only two steps. But a lot of frustrating/discouraging things can happen in a new gym that may make you falsely conclude that working out is too hard and embarrassing before you ever accomplish the working-out part. This is especially true if your time is limited.

So: the important thing here is to go in with zero expectation of doing all the reps and sets you have programmed for yourself, or maybe even of sorting out all the logistics, *at first*. You are basically doing a dry run. All you're doing in this session is figuring out:

- where the stuff you need actually is (appropriately sized dumbbells, squat racks, deadlift platforms, clips)
- roughly how to use it
- any of the soft interactions you need to do in order to use it (asking to work in, asking for next, asking the gym staff how some piece of equipment works)

Basically, this means you will find the equipment, get to the point of being all set up to use it and have everything you need, and stop short of expecting to have the time and patience to do all your sets and reps.

For instance, with squats you will:

- find the squat rack
- ask the person using it how many sets they have left
- take command of it
- set it to the right height and find the clips
- locate all the right plates that you need (2.5s, 5s, 10s, 25s)
- make sure the safety arms on either side aren't too high or too low for you when you squat
- maybe figure out where you can set up a camera to film your sets

And that's it. Technically, you can walk away at that point. (It might feel weird, but again, no one is really paying attention to what anyone else is doing.) If all that ended up being perfectly breezy and you want to do a set or two, or all your sets, with the empty bar or with more weight, that's also totally fine. Then you'll go to your next movement and do the same process.

This may end up taking way less time than an actual workout, if everything is easy. It might take up as much time or a little longer. Don't take that to mean actually working out will take *even longer* than that; it will not. It'll all flow smoother the next time, and the time after that. If you don't get to everything, or have a second "day" of training to figure out, like your Days A and B in this program, by all means, do this a second time. People take all kinds of pre-production non-work seriously; whole jobs are structured around essentially going on vacation to see if it would be nice to film a movie there ("location scouting").

So once you've done this, hopefully (a) it didn't ultimately take more than a week or so of your time, and (b) you are feeling ready to put all the pieces together for the next step—step three: Actually Doing Your Workout.

HOW TO START GOING TO THE GYM, PART 3: HOW MUCH WEIGHT TO USE

Finally here we are at part three of "starting to go to the gym," whether you are a complete noob, a seasoned intermediate exploring a new gym for the first time, or dialing back in after a long break. Now that you have scoped out the gym for vibes in part one, and given yourself some space and time to do basic recon on how all the equipment works in part two, it's time to actually touch weights.

However, this is the point where people roll up to the deadlift platform/squat rack/dumbbell rack/lat pulldown machine, the light of God upon their heads, the Kygo remix of "Higher Love" in their hearts, only to stand astride the equipment and go:

"Ah fuck; I have no idea how much weight to use. This has now made me so nervous I also forget how to do the movement that I so assiduously practiced at home. Oh no; oh no; uhhh," *nervously does some dumbbell curls and goes home*

We've all been there. Don't worry; I got you!

There is a basic truth to begin from here: With or without a training background, people can be all different levels and types of strong. Some people can step up to the squat rack and squat a plate (135lbs) their first go. Some people may have been bodily carrying a few baby-to-toddler-age kids around for a few years and can bench 75lbs without breaking a sweat. Many (most) people will be able to do less than this. All of these beginning points are fine.

So where to actually, numerically start? Here is the process:

- Ten pounds (or two 5lb dumbbells) will be a good place to start for any lift, if you are totally in the dark. You may find ten pounds is plenty, and then that becomes your first ever working weight. You can then count that first set as a working set, do the rest of your sets, and move on.
- If ten pounds is easy (like you do the number of prescribed working-set reps as a test, and find you could immediately go again), go up to 15 or 20 pounds.
- If that's still really, really easy, go up to 30 or 40 pounds. Keep going and adding weight like this. Rest a minute if you do several sets in a row and are feeling a little tired out by all this experimentation.
- Most people for any lift are not going to be able to add weight like this more than a few times. If you can: Congrats! You are surprisingly strong. But if you find your challenging weight quickly: Stop! Rest a minute. After that, do your working sets with your newly found working weight if you feel like it, or move on to the next movement in your session.

> If you overshoot (say you jump from 30 to 40, and 30 felt too easy but 40 makes you crumple to the ground instantly and you can't even do one rep): Stop. Rest a minute. Then do your working sets with your newly found working weight (in this example, 30 or 35 pounds), or move on.

A key element here is that, even if you start with a weight that is too easy, the magic of linear progression means you are going to be adding weight the very next session. You can add as little as 2.5lbs, but you can add 10lbs or more if you're able. This means the weights get to be no joke pretty fast, even if they start out joke-adjacent! You can just find a weight that feels easy enough and linearly progress from there. I promise it will get challenging pretty quickly.

If you are doing, say, ten sets before you feel like you find an appropriate working weight—say you were playing it really safe adding only 2.5lbs at a time, but you've done ten sets and only worked your way from 10 pounds to 35 pounds and it still doesn't feel challenging—you will be SOME kind of sapped from all that extra legwork. Then it feels a bit unfair when you "find a working weight," because your working weight may not be as much as you are capable of as if you had been able to dial it in several sets ago.

But still, that weight is unlikely to be SO far off that you could actually be doing, say, double or triple what it is. You might be off by 5, 10, 20 pounds. That's not that much, in the grand scheme. If you are following linear progression and adding 2.5-10lbs per lift, you would be finding your way to that higher weight in just a few sessions. This is nothing to stress over.

Once you've done this, congrats! You have fully smoothed the groove with your new gym and your new routine, and you are prepared to start lifting in earnest. Things may still go wrong, but like going to any new place, you need room to gain experience with this new environment. I've started over at or visited many new gyms, and they are not all as similar or as intuitive as you might think. It's not you! Just be patient with yourself and this new place, and it's all going to be okay.

RECORDING YOUR WORKOUTS

YOUR LIFTING NOTEBOOK

There is space in the LIFTOFF templates to record how your workout went. And you should use it. You think you will remember how things felt or what you did last time, but we have too many things on our minds to remember what squatting felt like two days ago. Take that pressure off of your brain.

You should record not only the weight you lifted, but how it felt, and what issues you had, if any. You can write down if you failed a set, so you know to back off the weight next time (or to check if your period is coming, and is maybe making you tired!) If you like, you can rate how you felt that day out of 5, or 10. This can be as intensive or simple as you want; the only real rule is to record the weight you lifted that day and whether you completed your sets.

These notes will also help you learn to view any issues you have, not as personal shortcomings, but data that you can manage. Whatever problem you have, I assure you someone has had it before and there is a way to address it. You are not the first person on earth to feel like you're falling forward in your squat, or like your bench gets stuck if you actually lower the barbell all the way to your chest, or like you feel deadlifts only in your lower back. These are all eminently fixable issues, and you can't begin to address them if you don't acknowledge that they're happening and make a plan to find out what's going on.

In Phase One, when you aren't using weights yet, make notes on your form and how various movements feel. Was your squat to depth? Did you feel your hip hinge only in your lower back still? Were your pushups so easy that you're now ready to move to a lower surface in your incline pushups?

In Phases Two and Three, you will start to record the weights you lifted per movement, and can keep recording more qualitative observations about how the lifts felt. Did you feel like you did nothing at all, or did you feel like you were about to faint? Were you falling forward or backward in your squats? Did you fail a lift and now you need to deload next session?

Not only will this allow you to look back on your ~memories~ of the days you started lifting, but you will be able to see how far you came. "Seeing how far you came" is maybe the single most important aspect of this whole thing. If you prefer, you can copy down the workouts into a notebook and keep track of your feelings and weights there (this is what I do; yes it's a composition notebook a la Harriet the Spy; no I won't be taking further questions). My notes extend from "AHHH IT FELT GREAT!! Go up in weight next time" to "PMS :(" to "Had to stop workout; squirrel got in the house." These notes are useful not just for the next session, but to see how your workouts are going overall and to notice trends. For instance, if squirrels are too regularly disrupting your workouts, perhaps something should be done about that.

TAKING VIDEO OF YOUR LIFTS

I know recording video of your lifts feels so conspicuous and embarrassing to someone who is not the Big Man on Campus in the weight room. But look: We can't improve what we can't measure, and the only way to measure form is for you (and other people) to see it. Watching in a mirror is not the same, and is even specifically inadvisable, because the angle at which you will naturally be looking during a lift is not the right angle to actually observe any lift. The mirrors in gyms are for people to admire their muscles, not to check form. You will get so much more information being able to see yourself from the perspective of a third person.

Therefore: use your phone to record yourself lifting from various non-mirror angles, and compare and contrast to the instructional videos. (If you are a paying subscriber to the She's A Beast newsletter, there is a #form-check channel where you can get feedback from other lifters.) You can also post them to the #couchobarbell hashtag to share your lifting journey and help show that no one has to be an Olympian to try out, and enjoy, strength training.

Not unlike your personal lifting notebook, I promise you will treasure your early lifting videos. I didn't ever record myself in my early lifting days, and I completely regret it!! I SO wish I could see how much I actually improved, but I was too big of a scaredy baby to set my phone up on the gym floor for 30 whole seconds to capture my squat sets, and now those moments are lost to time. Don't be like me.

You don't even need a fancy little tripod. Prop your phone up with a water bottle or an extra shoe or even some spare plates (if you lie two plates on the floor and wedge your phone between them, it will stand up straight).

FAILING, AND GETTING A SPOTTER

Oh no—you failed!

In real life, "failure" can have extremely dire implications. But in lifting, it's just the term for "not being able to complete your intended reps for the set." Maybe you had to drop the weight on the floor, or let it fall to the safety racks.

Failing feels absolutely humiliating the first time it happens. But since you're a newb (no offense) I want you to believe me here: In this place, failing is the most normal thing in the world. Provided no one is in imminent danger, experienced lifters do not even bat an eyelash at someone failing their lift.

Failure is part of growth. If you never fail, you're probably holding back. People who fail are the people who were willing try and risk not succeeding. In the choice between being a scaredy-cat and being a failure, you should pick "failure," maybe not every time, but at least SOME of the time, just as a check on whether you might be shortchanging your progress.

Failing with a barbell is tricky only during benching and squatting. During bench, when we are dealing with lower weights, you can simply drop it to your chest and roll it down your body, or dump the weights off either side (don't use clips, if you are anticipating that scenario). With squats, it's better for the weight to fall backwards past your butt than forward over your head, for obvious reasons.

So what do you do when it happens?

- Accept help from anyone who is offering (e.g. helping to lift the barbell off your chest, in the case of bench)
- Thank them
- Unload the barbell
- Put the barbell back on its pegs
- Reload the barbell

Ideally, you should prevent the worst of the failure scenarios by asking someone in your gym to spot you. Getting a spotter (someone to supervise your lift and help you bail if it goes awry) is another thing that will help you avoid Scaredy-Cat Mode (SCM) and allow you to challenge yourself, knowing that someone is there you help you. Once again, asking for a spot sounds and feels absolutely humiliating to a newb, but in this case, too: most normal thing in the world to experienced lifters.

This interaction goes like so: When you're ready to lift, find someone who is working out nearby you, maybe resting between sets, and say "Hey, can you spot me?" When they say "Sure!" and follow you over, let them know how many reps you are attempting (so they can have an idea of when you are getting to the point when you might need help), plus any special instructions (I like to tell them "Don't touch the bar unless there is downward motion"). Thank them afterward. And be a good citizen of the gym; be a willing spottee as well.

RECOVERY, OR "EATING AND RESTING"

"Recovery" is everything you do outside the gym to take care of yourself: eating, sleeping, stretching, managing stress. Another oversight of the "workout"-based type of exercise is that it does not teach us to care at all about this stuff. If you're like me, you might have even been conditioned to believe, for instance, that eating a nice big meal after a workout would be "wasting the workout." In reality, the *opposite* is true: If you don't eat enough, you are only setting yourself up for an unfair and unnecessary amount of soreness. And this is true of all recovery dimensions: if you don't sleep, or if you don't manage your stress, you will be miserable trying to build muscle. This is how to manage your recovery.

EATING: EAT YOUR FOOD

Look at me in my two eyes: There is almost no point to working out if you don't eat properly to support it. This sounds like a bold statement, but if you've ever tried to crash-diet and go nuts working out at the same time, only to have everything fall apart and regain whatever few pounds you might have managed to lose, you already know exactly what I mean.

Without getting too deep into things, your number one goal with this guide is to build strength and muscle and progress in the form of "weights go up." This happens very, very slowly in the best of circumstances, to the tune of one pound per month for women, and maybe double that for men. And it only happens IF you are eating enough calories for your body to maintain your body weight.[1]

To create the best of "weights go up" circumstances, you need to make sure you are 1) training hard, and 2) fueling yourself properly. That means not only eating your protein, which supports rebuilding the muscles you broke down by working out, but eating the carbs and fats you need to fuel your workouts and your life. Take it from someone who spent all of her adult life wielding food like a weapon at herself: Food is for supporting your livelihood, not for torturing yourself.

---

1. If you try to eat less, your body won't be able to build your muscles and fuel your workouts, and you'll just stay in the same place you are. Addressing disordered eating is beyond the scope of LIFTOFF. But your experience, and your results, frankly, will be significantly impoverished if disordered eating behaviors or body dysmorphia to lord over your approach to this program. I've seen it too many times. Please trust me: You need your food.

When this 12 weeks is over, you can go on to wreak whatever havoc you wish upon your person, but while I have you, give this idea and process some room to work. You might think I'm being really intense about this, but it's so hard for me to watch someone get excited about lifting, only to shy away from the eating part and hold themselves to a meager 1,500 calories a day, which causes the whole experiment to founder. It's hard for them, too. Don't do that to yourself! If you struggle with this, it is a worthy reason to seek help from your favorite therapist or medical professional.

What happens if you don't eat? You will be very sore, way more sore than even my worst enemies deserve; and you will even potentially cause your body to eat away at your muscles, rather than protect and slowly cultivate them.

This is not a weight-loss program. However, the process of starting strength training and building muscles in most people triggers a process called "recomposition." When your body is in recomposition, it is building muscle and losing body fat at the same time. You stay about the same weight, but may become a little physically smaller. See the "What's going to happen to your body" section for diagrams explaining this.

So how do you know how much food is the right amount? On a personal note, as someone whose nutritional education was virtually sideways when I started lifting, tracking my calories and macros was absolutely critical for learning what "enough protein" looked like, what the proteinful foods were, whether I was eating enough carbs to fuel my workouts, and many other things. Tracking food has gotten a bad rap recently, which feels a bit unfair, because a dirty secret of many "intuitive eaters" online who do strength training is that they are able to "eat intuitively" because they spent a long time tracking their foods, and have a lot of practice at putting together balanced meals. This did not come naturally to someone like myself, who was disappointed to find my usual meal of "a bowl of cereal" had only like 7 grams of protein, and then I had to scramble to figure out what else to eat to get the other 133 grams.

Tracking food is certainly not required for this program. If you can't tolerate food numbers, skip to the Resting section below, and know that all you have to really do here is "eat a lot" and "eat a lot of protein" (a palm's worth or two per meal, and more if you need. You "need" more protein when your weights are not going up). You are not "eating a lot" for the rest of your life, you're only doing it for the duration of this program. That can be the whole game. If your progress suffers, not eating enough food and protein is usually the issue, followed by "not great-enough form."

Here is how to get started with basic tracking: Calculate your total daily energy expenditure, or TDEE, using your current height, weight, age, gender (for scientific purposes, this calculator is pre-set at an activity level of "some"; that is, not "none" and not "professional athlete doing two-a-days." "Some" activity is consistent with the three-days-a-week structure of LIFTOFF, plus a bit of recovery activity if you feel like it). This will tell you is roughly how many calories you should be eating in a day. The equations below are designed for people who are building muscle while holding their body weight steady, balancing their energy input and output.

For men, your TDEE for building muscle = (66+(13.7*
[your body weight in pounds]/2.204)+(5***[your height in inches]**2.54)-(6.8***[your age in years]**))*1.55.

For women, your TDEE for building muscle = (665+(9.6*
[your body weight in pounds]/2.204)+(1.8***[your height in inches]**2.54)-(4.7***[your age in years]**))*1.55

Out of those calories, aim for your protein intake to be 1 gram per pound of body weight. (Technically, ~technically~, you can get away with .82 grams per pound of body weight, according to research. But I personally feel and notice a difference trying to get slightly more protein, whether that's because I under-measure; I am genetically feeble and synthesize protein badly; or some other reason. Feel free to try this lower number, but if you don't see the harmonious progress you should be seeing, know that I am somewhere, wiggling my eyebrows at you.)

The science around precise protein intake is a bit fuzzy and depends on a lot of factors. Protein is less widely available or present in as many foods as carbs or fat. Because of that and a few other reasons, it's prohibitively hard to consume TOO MUCH protein. That's a big reason to err on the high end.

If you have body fat over 30 percent of your body weight (this is likely if you have a minimal training/athletic background and your BMI is >30), you can scale down to 1 gram per pound of lean body mass (so that would be your body weight * 0.7). If you aren't sure what your body fat percentage is, try eating the smaller amount of protein, and go up if your weights aren't progressing. Or do the reverse: Eat the higher amount and see what happens if you scale it back a bit.

You should also favor whole-foods-style proteins over, say, several scoops of protein powder per day (that said, a scoop of protein powder can go a long way toward closing the gap left by meals). Food is complex, micronutrients matter, so don't try to do much high-wire engineering with vitamins and supplements and so forth. Eat real food if you can, but a scoop of protein won't hurt you, the end.

Example: a 30-year-old, 150-pound, 5'4" woman has a TDEE of 2,082 calories per day. She should aim to eat 120-150 grams of protein per day (480-600 calories), which means she has about 1,482 calories remaining to divvy up between fats and carbs. If she suspected she was over 30 percent body fat, she could try starting with 105 grams of protein, and increase it if she feels bad in the gym and her weights are not progressing as they should.

An important thing to keep in mind is that, while we can calculate calories and grams down to single digits, your body has a lot of processes for smoothing out some "noise" in your energy input and output, so to speak (read about NEAT, if you've never heard of it before). An extra gram here or there or 50 or 70 calories is nothing to stress over. It's best to think of your food intake as it pertains to your lifting progress on a week-to-week basis, as opposed to meal to meal or day to day. Your gains aren't lost if you don't guzzle 40 grams of protein immediately after your workout, and you're not fucked for your workout tomorrow because you had some pizza and beer instead of a boiled chicken breast and broccoli. You will be in a largely good place making sure you are fueled pretty evenly throughout the day and week.

Depending on your personal biology and metabolism, you may need to eat a little bit more or less than what the TDEE figure says. It may help to keep in mind what you've been eating when you have your next gym session, and record in your notebook if a particular amount of food helped you feel good or bad.

It's good to keep in mind in general that TDEE and protein intake are suggestions, not rules. Some people will need a little more of either or both, or may be able to get away with less (but not radically so; we're talking like a 20% difference, not 50% or 100%). It's not a bad thing to experiment a little with your own numbers, to see if more helps, or to see if you're fine with less. But if your weights aren't going up, and you haven't looked more closely at your food numbers, you know why.

However, I have to stress that everything balances out according to the Avocado Principle from earlier *only under the conditions that you are progressing your weights, going to the gym regularly, and getting enough protein as well as carbs and fats to make that happen.*

Sometimes, people undereat by a little, hoping to cheat the system and get stronger but also lose a bit of body weight. It not only doesn't work that way, but it can kind of cause the whole project to unravel, such that the person doesn't progress, but also gains weight. Yes, really! Not that there's anything wrong with that, but it can happen!

Sometimes, people start eating everything in sight, but still aren't getting enough protein, and also aren't methodically making their weights go up. This, also, violates the Avocado Principle covenant. There's nothing wrong with this either! But I can't promise an outcome if you are futzing around with the inputs.

In the same vein, if you are doing LIFTOFF but choosing not to participate in the "weights go up" part, that is completely fine as well. But this does not meet the criteria for recomposition. Recomposition doesn't happen magically because you pick up some dumbbells for a bit a few times a week, unfortunately. That is why I have tried to be quite clear about the circumstances that produce it.

I focus on recomposition because it's the middle of the road approach for most people, and it'll hold you, as a variable, steady so you can appreciate and enjoy these changes and challenges. If recomposition is not your goal, there are too many variables for me help further with what to eat or how to achieve their desired results via this book, but a dietitian or lifting coach can be very helpful!

Drink your water, too; 11.5 cups of fluids for women and 15.5 cups for men per day.

If you aren't sure what the whole picture of what you eat should look like with that much protein, Eat This Much is an extremely useful site. Some high-protein sources of food that I like: pretty much any meat, vegetarian substitute meats, eggs, Greek yogurt, string cheese, tinned fish, cottage cheese, turkey pepperoni, protein powder, edamame, tofu.

There are a lot of foods that many people think are "high in protein" that are not, such as peanut butter. A tracking app can be useful to set yourself straight in this matter, such as Cronometer, MyFitnessPal, or MacroFactor. Turn off any built-in goal-setting garbage and set your own caloric intake and macro (protein/fat/carbs) goal numbers. I will use apps like this because they help me to make sure I'm eating *enough* of the things I need, and they allow me to experiment and tweak servings to dial in the right amounts; for instance, why eat 7 ounces of chicken if can get away with 5 ounces and then eat two eggs later?

If you are interested in more reading on the topic of nutrition, Renaissance Woman/Renaissance Diet 2.0 are the best books I've read on this subject. The r/xxfitness subreddit also has a nice nutrition FAQ. For food and recipe ideas, refer to Eat This Much, Fit Men Cook, and Meal Prep Manual. Links to all of these resources may be found in the Resources section.

RESTING: SLEEP 7-9 HOURS, MINIMIZE OTHER ACTIVITY ENOUGH TO SUPPORT "WEIGHTS GO UP"

You know how plants grow with sunlight and water, but if you were to put most plants in 24 hours of sun and dump several gallons of water on them a day, they would die? You are the plant in this scenario, and the sun is "working out"; your body likes good things, but even with good things, your body can only take so much.

The three-days-a-week structure of LIFTOFF doesn't just mean "work out three days a week"; it also means "don't work out strenuously the rest of the days of that week." It's important that you give yourself a chance to understand the full scope of the strength-building feedback loop, and that won't happen if you are piling in a bunch of other activities, AND ALSO trying to lose 10 pounds, AND ALSO trying to run a marathon. Stop—stop—stop. I'm writing you a metaphorical permission slip to stop. Just give yourself a chance here.

How much is too much? "Too much" is whatever causes your form to suffer and your progress to slow. If you're still able to add weight predictably to your lifts, *and* train for a marathon? God bless you, you genetic freak, I don't know what you are doing here when you could be playing in the NBA. But for 99.99% of us, that won't happen. As I've said elsewhere, you may go nuts on yourself on your own time, but within this program, I ask you to locate inner peace and give this space to work. If you are doing "other stuff" and are the weights aren't going up 2.5-5lbs every session, guess what you need to stop doing, or at least strive to do less of? That's right—other stuff.

All that said: 20 minutes of light cardio such as walking, or some gentle yoga, won't kill your gains, and might even help if you are sore. If you either enjoy it, want to try it, or feel like it might help your lifting journey, diversifying your activity a bit won't kill you. If you don't move much in your daily life otherwise, it would be fine to aim to get in 5,000 or so steps a day, or 20ish minutes of other gentle activity. If you absolutely must do something more moderate-intensity, like HIIT or running or playing sports, try to keep it under an hour once a week, ideally with a rest day after.

If you are struggling with the form for any of the lifts and hitting mobility limitations, try to do some mobility work on your rest days. See the "A note on squat depth" section. For the other lifts, simply practicing the movement should help a lot, and the same goes for some basic stretching.

Not only should you be conserving your energy to a reasonable degree, but you should be prioritizing your sleep. You need good quality sleep for 7-9 hours. Try to lighten up on the alcohol if you tend to drink a lot (too much all the time interferes with your muscles' ability to recover); have some weed instead, honestly. Manage your personal stress as best as you are able.

If you feel bad or injured, refer to the relevant FAQs in the FAQs section. But generally, remember: 80% or even 60% is better than nothing, if you are able. If you are not able: All of this is about taking care of your health, and sometimes that takes the form of accepting the changes of "what progress looks like." When you are injured, progress becomes "recovering fully so you can get back to lifting."

WHAT TO DO IF WEIGHTS WON'T GO UP

(AND A NOTE ABOUT OHP)

Okay, look; overhead press can be a bitch. It's so hard. It's almost universally the first lift on which you will stall, or fail and then not be able to add weight, because of the body position it requires and because the muscles it uses are so small. Fortunately, there are a number of ways you can deal with this. You may also stall at some points on other lifts; this is normal and okay, you are not the first person for this to happen to, and you can overcome!

The first way to deal is to be spot-on with your form. You might be saying, "But Casey, I know how to lift things above my head." No disrespect to you, but I bet you don't! I bet you are not using your lats, and your elbows are all akimbo. It's okay; we and I were all like this at some point. But your body is never going to get strong at moving that way if you don't dial in the right movement pattern. Humble yourself before what you might think is just a simplistic "wave your arms in the air like you just don't care" motion. It's a little trickier than you think, but worth getting right,

It's possible that you can overhead-press more weight right now doing it the way you are used to doing it, instead of the way you are supposed to do it. Maybe you can do 5 reps of 50 pounds doing it your way, and only 5 reps of 30 pounds the "right" way. But when we lift more weight at the expense of form, functionality, and sanity, it's called "ego lifting." Don't do it. Who are we, or you, trying to impress? And to be honest, whoever it is probably won't be impressed by 20 extra pounds.

Even with good form, you will probably stall first on overhead press before any other lift. But you can stall on any lift at any time, for lots of different reasons. This is how to deal with stalling. You can use this approach for ANY lift you stall on.

If you're sure your form is on point, the way to deal with stalling is to go up each session in smaller increments. Instead of adding 2.5 pounds for the next session, add one pound, or even half a pound, if you have access to plates that small.

If very small increment plates aren't available, here's what you're going to do: rep-based progressive overload, or "reps go up."

Go back down to the last weight increment you could successfully do, *with good form*. Now instead of doing 3 sets of 5 reps, you'll do 2 sets of 5 reps, and then a third set with one more rep than the previous session. Like so:

Session 1: 2x5, and then 1x6 as a last set
Session 2: 2x5, and then 1x7 as a last set
Session 3: 2x5, and then 1x8 as a last set
Session 4: 2x5, and then 1x9 as a last set
Session 5: 2x5, and then 1x10 as a last set
Session 6: 3x5 with the next weight increment up

This is about as slow as you can progress and not be going backward. But it's still progress! You might even be able to go a little faster (7 reps on the last set one session, then 9 the next session, and then be ready to do the next weight increment up the session after that). You could also speed it up by adding one rep per set, so you do 3x5 one session, 3x6 the next, 3x7 the next, then 3x8. At that point, you should attempt the next weight up again. But the general point is to focus on accumulating more reps across all your sets with each additional session, until you can onramp yourself to the next weight.

Lastly, if you stall on OHP specifically before the program is over, but you are able to do 3 sets of 5 with about half your body weight, you've been adding weight so fast that you're probably pretty close to topping out in a linear progression program like this anyway. So just keep doing the reps you can do until the program is over.

A NOTE ON DEADLIFTS

So you have made it through all of the hip hinges and RDLs, and are finally ready to take a stab at conventional deadlifts. That's great! I'm terrible at deadlifts, but they are one of my favorite lifts to train.

When you are learning to deadlift, the barbell should be about 8.5 inches off the floor. The problem is, if you do not have access to bumper plates (plates that are the same size as regular 45lb plates, but lighter) and can't yet lift a barbell with 45 pounds loaded on each end (135lbs total), the barbell lying on the floor will be positioned significantly lower than that. This is a problem, because as you may have noticed in the form videos, deadlift setups are based on orienting yourself around the barbell at that height. If the barbell is off, you are off.

Well, shit. Welcome to "a problem that gave me enormous trouble while I was trying to learn to lift."

So here are your options:

Keep using dumbbells, or even fixed barbells, to do RDLs for a while. You will probably have to reset to a lower weight once you move to doing conventional deadlifts, because it has a longer range of motion and uses new muscles.

But you don't have to jump to using a full-size barbell as soon as you cross the 45lb RDL threshold, either. As long as you're able to maneuver the dumbbells and/or fixed barbells, you can keep doing RDLs with them, on the idea that it will carry over to deadlifts; i.e., if you can get up to doing a 90lb RDL, you will probably be able to start your deadlifts with 65 or 75lbs, instead of 45lbs.

But! You will probably NOT be able to make it all the way to 135lbs of RDL and then seamlessly transition to a 135lb deadlift. So when that moment comes, here are the rest of your options:

Use risers, mats, piles of books, piles of plates, anything that can get the barbell up to about the right height. It doesn't have to be perfect, but it should be close. If you have a standard iron 25lb plate loaded on either end, two 25lb plates laid on the floor stacked on top of each other under both ends should get you pretty close. That's a lot of 25lb plates to be hoarding and moving around, but bear in mind you will soon progress beyond this, and you don't have to do it forever.

Beg the gym to buy a set of bumper plates, or buy your own, and maybe ask the gym to store them for you. This is an investment that, in my opinion, gyms should want to make. A pair of 10lb bumper plates is $60, and those will be sturdy enough to load to bridge the gap to 135 pounds. In my imagination, you'd also be able to buy your own set and keep them in your car and bring them in to use, inspiring "who is she" whispers of admiration throughout the weight room. I could see this being a liability issue, somehow, but it feels worth asking if it would be allowed!

Do a "deficit deadlift" and lift from the floor as best you can. Technically a too-low deadlift is still a deadlift, it's just a special variety called a "deficit deadlift." This is your best option if you are too embarrassed to do any of these other options. Because the range of motion is longer, the lift will be slightly harder than it needs to be (and you will need more mobility than you would for a standard-height deadlift, and for this period of time you won't be dialing in your actual deadlift form as much as you could be). But you only need to grit through this until you get to 135lbs, which should be fairly quick and straightforward, because deadlifts use all the biggest muscles in your body.

You'll have to relearn form a bit once you get to regulation-size plates, but this isn't the end of the world. You should set up with the same cues: barbell over mid-foot, and push your hips out/bend at the knees to bring your shins to the barbell as you grab onto it.

Try to approximate the height with just your movement. This is the least desirable option, but it's essentially what I did, and while I don't think I had a model deadlift education, I did live to tell this tale. During the part of the rep where you lower the weight back to the floor instead of going all the way back down, just pause and reverse when the bar gets to your mid-shin. This is your best option if you can't get into a good position mobility-wise to do the deficit deadlifts. Your form will also probably suffer because you can't set up correctly around the stationary barbell on the floor, and are instead making a lot of guesses as you where your knees, hips, shoulders, and torso should be as you go down and back up. Please at least strongly consider one of the other options before doing this.

A NOTE ON SQUAT DEPTH

People squat to below parallel (hip crease below the top of the knee) for two reasons:

1. Your body uses slightly different (and important!) muscles as you go from an above-parallel squat to a below-parallel squat; you can above-parallel-squat using almost entirely your quads, but a good below-parallel squat requires your body to at least begin thinking about your glutes and hamstrings. Your body also needs good range of motion to get below parallel in a way that it doesn't as much for above parallel.
2. It is the only way to do a complete and legal squat within the sport of powerlifting in some federations.

We are mostly concerned with the first point, here. The thing about squat depth is that many people just getting started with lifting will often "skip" it, often out of fear or discouragement. This can lead to a snowballing effect where their squat becomes higher and higher as they add weight, and their fear about hitting depth grows and grows, and their squat becomes less and less of a functional, strength-building movement. Obviously, neither I nor the police are going to show up and arrest you if your squat is not quite below parallel. But as someone who wants to help you develop good body movement above all else, I care that you care about getting decent squat depth.

Most people, particularly sedentary people, will struggle with squat depth. This is normal and okay, because it's a skill you can develop. There are three good ways of doing this:

1. Hang out in the lowest squat position you can manage with good form/without back rounding or hyperextending/arching. You will probably feel all different muscles stretching when you do this, and this will help develop stability as well as mobility. If you feel like you're falling backward or forward as your get lower in the squat, to the point that you can't reach full depth—this is a very common issue! Practice squatting while you holding an upright like the side of a door, a door frame, a stair banister or a box right in front of you. Practice resting at the lowest level you can with good form, back flat and straight and heels on the floor, to help teach your muscles to work together, stretch them, and build your depth. As you build your depth, practice releasing your grip on the support in front of you more and more, until you are able to rest in the bottom of your squat with no support. Hold for 3 sets of 30 seconds or as long as you can.
2. Work on general mobility. Try doing a regular, short stretching routine (seriously five minutes) daily. You are in a situation where probably anything will help. But one stretch that can be super-helpful to squatting is the frog stretch: get down on all fours, then slide your knees away from each other in a split position, until it's slightly uncomfortable. Lower yourself on your arms

to your elbows, and rest in this position. If you can, try rocking back gently into your hips. Just holding this position with light tension for 15-30 seconds can help build better squat positioning.

DOES THIS MEAN I SHOULD SQUAT AS LOW AS HUMANLY POSSIBLE?

No. There are diminishing returns and significant potential downsides to "ass to grass" squatting, particularly that it can cause many people to lose all tension and try to bounce their whole body weight off their calves and knee joints, which does not a strong and resilient and mechanically sound body make. It also requires increasingly good mobility to get really, really low without form compromises like butt winking/back rounding (no need to worry intensively about those right now, but if you keep going with lifting beyond LIFTOFF, they will be something to look into). I will be more than satisfied by a nice, obviously-below-parallel-but-not-wildly-more-than-that squat.

DOES THIS MEAN "DON'T PROGRESS IN YOUR SQUAT UNTIL YOU ARE ABLE TO GET BELOW PARALLEL?"

Also no. The scenario we are trying to avoid is "fear of developing squat depth because going any deeper than you currently can feels scary." It may take weeks or months before you develop really good mobility, and the weights in LIFTOFF are not going up SO fast that you can't walk and chew bubblegum at the same time here (that is, build your strength AND develop mobility). Just don't forego either at the expense of the other. If you notice your squat is getting higher and higher as you add weight, back your progress up a little (see the "What to do if you stall" section) and do your best to re-calibrate your depth before moving on.

If you end LIFTOFF with a squat that is high, that's not the end of the world. But from there, I would strongly suggest putting in some work on depth!

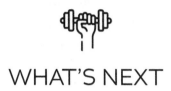

WHAT'S NEXT

Well would you look at that—12 weeks flew by, and now LIFTOFF is over!!

By this time, you should be able to handle a barbell more than capably, as well as plates and racks. You are probably well on your way to squatting or deadlifting the equivalent of your body weight. Not only that, but you are probably noticing changes in your body, and I don't just mean the new muscle definition shadows in the locker room mirror—you're moving differently, too. You feel strong. You feel capable. When you push or pull or bend or lean over, you don't feel sad and ineffectual, or like you're about to fall over; you feel powerful, like Wonder Woman or King Kong. Congrats! That was exactly the idea this whole time.

But hold on; we went through this whole journey together, and now I'm just going to leave you? Well, yes, but also, only sort of; you have a lot of options from here.

IF... YOU'RE NOT READY FOR THIS TO BE OVER!

Time for a special surprise: You can keep doing Phase Three of LIFTOFF for quite a bit longer. This is a linear progression program, and for someone who is working hard, recovering well, and making steady progress, about six total months of good progress (maybe more!) will go by from the time they started LIFTOFF before they even really need to start thinking about changing up their programming. Share your progress with the #couchtobarbell hashtag so that others can see what real people doing strength training looks like.

By the end of LIFTOFF, you might have zeroed in on some of your personal areas of improvement, or new desired strength goals. You might be interested in more specifically training to get your pull-up, for example, or maybe you have realized your hamstrings are just not getting with the program, and you could stand more hamstring-oriented accessories to get them up to speed. It should be possible to add specific accessories to LIFTOFF to meet your goals, but that's your own personal journey, and I truly wish you luck and happiness on it. Maybe someday I will get around to making a LIFTOFF+ that accommodates this. But in the meantime, GZCLP is a good and very similar-to-LIFTOFF programming option for those who want a linear progression program they can customize.

The real, meaningful end to a linear progression program comes when you can't continue to add weight every session, provided that your form, recovery, and consistency are all good (you can check a strength standards chart for reference, but being able to lift 0.25 x bodyweight OHP, 0.5x bench, 1x squat, and 1.5x deadlift are decent rules of thumb for "the end of beginner gains"). At that point, you would move to a more novice-intermediate format, where your weight increases will happen in periods of weeks, not days/sessions (this is more like how GZCLP works).

When you get to that intermediate point, there are a ton of free options; GZCL, 5/3/1, PHUL, and PPL are four tried and true ones. A program called Tactical Barbell is very popular with a bunch of my newsletter subscribers. Lots of trainers offer barbell programming for subscription fees. Go have fun. If you want to get a lot stronger, you might consider a more hypertrophy-oriented program (that will probably look like more movements per workout, with lots of sets of 8-12 reps). There are two whole She's A Beast column for paid subscribers you may find in the Resources section.

Likewise, if you'd like to do even more reading about lifting beyond this book, my newsletter, She's A Beast, has covered an enormous range of topics and questions from readers just like you. You can access the entire archive at shesabeast.co.

IF... YOU WANT TO SCALE BACK LIFTING A LITTLE TO MAKE ROOM FOR OTHER TRAINING/ACTIVITIES

If you just like lifting as a workout, you can stop trying to progress and just maintain your strength with the weights you're at. Coast a while, my friend. If you want to maintain, LIFTOFF is formatted such that you can switch to doing Day A and Day B once each per week, and that should keep you pretty on track. Scaling back to two days a week leaves more room for other activities. Keep at least one rest day between your days, if at all possible. If not, switch to doing all your lower-body moves one day, and all upper-body moves the next day.

You could also, at this point, seek out a strength program more directly suited to your sport and give that a shot; now that you have built some raw strength, you will probably be do harder things than before in your sport or in these more sport-specific workouts, and see better results.

IF... YOU WANT TO CHANGE YOUR BODY COMPOSITION SUBSTANTIALLY (I.E., LOSE A LOT OF BODY FAT OR GAIN SIGNIFICANT MUSCLE)

If you want to change your body composition, you honestly should keep lifting; there's a reason people who do that for a job (bodybuilders) all lift weights, but not all of them do cardio. This should be a beautiful and cherished period of your life where you don't have to do any particular diet manipulations, you can just eat and grow! If I were making a personal recommendation, I would say keep going with a linear progression until you hit the six-month mark, and/or when you come to the end of beginner gains (you can check a strength standards chart for reference, but being able to lift 0.25 x bodyweight OHP, 0.5x bench, 1x squat, and 1.5x deadlift are decent rules of thumb). At that point, the best thing to do would be to seek a professional like a dietitian or nutrition coach familiar with strength training who can help you figure out your next best move.

But here is my armchair opinion, *if body composition change is your goal (which it does not have to be!)*: Research shows that people with higher body fat can continue to build muscle, even at a caloric deficit. If you are over 30 percent body fat (or would roughly estimate that you are based on pictures or your BMI), that means you can operate at a (modest! Not extreme!) calorie deficit, and likely continue to progress with your training. If you do NOT have higher body fat, again in my opinion, the best option is to recomp as long as you continue to get stronger, and then bulk first before you think about trying to lose body fat

This is all technically beyond the scope of LIFTOFF and again, my opinion. But I'm weighing in mostly because I'm tired of seeing women who are 18 percent body fat with no muscle on them to speak of ask the Internet they should bulk or cut, and then a cavalcade of other women respond, "Well it depends what you want! Do you want to be [pitying face of concern] a huge whale, or do you want to be a beautiful swan like [insert latest fitness influencer telling people they can get abs in two weeks]?"

Again, my opinion, but a woman who is 18 percent body fat and no muscle who wants to change her body composition has no business cutting first. We all need to love ourselves more than forcing ourselves to always be smaller, or to be extremely lean all the time; this is a weird fake standard that has become too common because of social media. I love social media, but this particular thing needs to stop. Anyway, moving on.

IF… YOU WANT TO STOP LIFTING ENTIRELY

If you want to stop lifting entirely, and start or go back to windsurfing or pole-dancing or rock-climbing, sally forth and enjoy your newfound strength. I hope you will find that having put in this time with LIFTOFF has helped you move a bit differently, perhaps with a little more pop, maybe a little more oomph. Maybe your mobility is better; maybe your agility is improved; maybe you're a little less breathless. If you switch activities, you may lose your gains a little more slowly than someone who doesn't do any kind of training at all.

Here is the thing: Muscle memory is real. I can't swear that you can stop working out entirely and keep feeling as capable as you do right now. But now that you've done this, it will always be easier to return to this point than it was to get here this first time. You made it through the strength woods, and you should be proud. If you ever wanted to come back from "not working out at all," you could simply run LIFTOFF all over again.

If you do a hard stop, you will probably backslide a bit. But that's okay. I thank you from the bottom of my heart for giving this a fair shot, and hope you got something significant out of it.

FAQS

> **Why are there only like six total movements? Why is there no core work? How can you have a strength training program in this century with no core work???**

There are only six total movements for simplicity. These six movements actually cover all the movement bases and basics of the human body (vertical pull, vertical push, horizontal pull, horizontal push).

And actually, there *is* core work: Your core is extremely activated any time you are moving free weights, because your body has to stabilize itself. That's why you use free weights and not Smith machines, bench machines, overhead press machines, etc.

When trainers have direct core work in their programs, it's likely because they feel pressure to include it. They feel pressure to include it because, despite all of us knowing that you can't spot-reduce body fat, a lot of people are self-conscious about their bellies and have been neuro-linguistic-programmed to believe that core work the only way to address that body fat, *and* that core work is our highest possible purpose as modern humans. Trainers are worried their programs won't be taken seriously without it.

I am not worried about that, because I know that this workout is already a good core workout, particularly for people who don't work out generally already, without movements that *only* work your core. I humbly redirect all further questions to my own abs.

> **This program looked and sounded boring, and now I've tried it, and it is boring. Am I doing something wrong?**

Possibly. This is not a "busywork" program meant to bamboozle you with hyperactivity. The "fun" or "challenge," so to speak, comes from the intensity and from getting to know your body.

There are two likely causes of your boredom: Your weights aren't heavy enough, or you're not getting and staying invested in your form and movement quality. Are you trying to use your muscles? Are you trying to hit squat depth? Are you buying into trying to actually challenge yourself with the 5-rep sets? Or are you just kind of, you know, doing them to check the box and then rolling your eyes for 60-90 seconds before doing them again?

I do not mean to be rude here, but you do have to give the "values" of this approach a chance, however skeptical you might be, if you expect it to also rise to the level of "fun" and "rewarding." If you can't do that, I sure can't promise you will feel anything or have any fun, and that is true also in life.

The beauty and difficulty of this program is in its simplicity. These compound movements both come to us naturally and have been discouraged or obscured by our daily lives. They are simple to learn, but hard to master. This isn't a program for someone who wants to just "feel busy"; it's a program for people who want to learn how to build, or rebuild, functionality in their body.

I've been lifting weights for several years now, and I'm still tweaking my squat, my bench, my deadlift. Perfecting these movements can be a lifelong journey, if you let it. But they don't have to be your lifelong journey; getting basically good at them can just be your short-term, limited-run journey.

The challenge is not just in the movements, but in the program. If it doesn't feel hard enough, use heavier weights. You'll know when they're hard enough when all you can do is kinda space out during the rest period until your next set.

If you're bored during your rests, you're almost definitely not working hard enough. If you're just bouncing on your joints through three sets of eight squats and calling it a day, you're doing it wrong. But if you're dialing in your mind-muscle connection and moving with intention, you're doing it right, and hopefully gathering data on what aspects aren't coming easily to you that you can focus on next time. That may not be everyone's perfect cup of tea, but is 12 weeks, 36 workouts, about 18 hours of time total, *so* much time to be a little bit bored?

Maybe this won't click for you even if you do give it a chance! Not everything is for everyone.

It is worth keeping in mind that working out is still working out, and taking care of yourself is still generally taking care of yourself. I don't like to clean my house or eat my vegetables and would rather sit immobile and watch TV all of my waking hours, but I work out at least in part because I'm trying to at least give myself a chance at stability, health, safety, and longevity. And frankly, I would actively feel pain in my body doing all that TV watching. I like my

TV-watching not interrupted by pain and discomfort, and working out helps with that.

> **My grip is barely strong enough to clamp/unclamp barbell clips. Do I have to use them?**

Again, the police won't show up, but it's nice to secure the plates so you don't have to worry about them wobbling or falling off as you lift. If your hands are too weak (been there!) one option is to buy, or ask your gym to buy, a set of barbell collars that lock and unlock and don't require grip strength to use. These can be found for pretty cheap now (around $10), are very worth the cost, and small enough to carry with you.

> **You said at the beginning that LIFTOFF was "compound movements with free weights," but the lat pulldown is a machine, is it not?**

Alright; no one likes a wise guy. You know if you insist on free-weight purity, you know you can do a pull-up progression instead of lat pulldowns? Don't chicken out now, Miss Strength Machine Hall Monitor :) You can see the recommended pull-up progression in the Resources section.

> **... Which way are the plates supposed to face on the barbell?? I see people doing both and don't want to look stupid.**

I face plates outward, so the writing is readable if you're standing at either end of the barbell. Most people face plates outward. I have noticed on the West Coast, for some reason, people have a slightly greater tendency to face them inward. Technically, in a powerlifting competition with nice plates, you face the first plate inward (so you can see it from the inside, I guess?), and the rest outward. Don't stress too much about this.

■ **My schedule doesn't allow for me to do three days a week every other day; I can do two days in a row, and then a third day one or two days later. Is that okay?**

It's not optimal, but try it! You should be super on-point with your recovery during those two-in-a-row days, eating lots of food, getting all your sleep, and probably not drinking or getting yourself involved in any stressful situations.

Another imaginative, though possibly bad, solution here would be to divide up the workouts on those days into lower-body one day (so, squats and then deadlifts) and upper body the next day (bench, overhead press, row, pull-ups/downs).

If neither of those things work, you could break up the days even further (one day on, two days off). It will hamper your gains, and I can't guarantee you'll get all the payoffs, but it's better than not trying at all. Bear in mind these workouts shouldn't take more than half an hour or so.

■ **Do I have to work out on the same days every week?**

No. As long as you're getting in three days a week with at least a day of rest in between, you are doing LIFTOFF exactly as intended. For other scenarios, refer to the other FAQs.

■ **My workouts are really, really long, longer than the estimated times given. What do I do?**

Having to wait for equipment, or having to rest an extended time between sets, can really inconveniently prolong your time in the gym. If you have to rest a REALLY long time between sets to feel ready for the next one, check in on your recovery; one minute of rest between sets at the pace of 2.5-5lbs per session shouldn't be a huge drag to accomplish.

If the equipment you need is scarce, you might need to do a bit of time management triage. For instance, right when you get to the gym, make contact with the person using the squat rack. Let them know you're just going to warm up quick and you'll be over there, and then go do your warm-up (nothing worse than warming up and then having to stand there for 15 minutes while someone wraps up!). Unless they are peaking for Nationals, they will be a lot closer to done by the time you're ready. If appropriate, warm up with dumbbells instead to the extent you can. (Good thing you learned all those dumbbell versions of the movements, too!)

Generally speaking, at a gym with only a couple of sets of whatever equipment you need, no one should be monopolizing them for the better part of an hour. If this is happening regularly, try talking to the gym staff and let them know you want to use the squat rack, but this jabroni has made camp in it, playing on his phone and doing curls for 45 minutes. The staff should be inspired to have a word with him about moving his curls elsewhere, or about being more conscientious of the ways in which he's infringing on other customers' livelihoods. Perhaps they will be moved to get a second or third rack, given all the customer interest!

Also, try just conspicuously standing nearby. Humans with hearts and brains will notice others are waiting.

You may not love this either, but just throwing out a suggestion: Try looking around for other gyms. Non-chain gyms are often not as crowded and can be very welcoming of people who love strength training, but may not advertise as well or pop up on Google Maps as aggressively. Non-chain gyms also, crucially, often don't require a membership commitment or have impossible-to-cancel contracts! They will let you pay for a month, or even a day, and that can be it. If your gym is chronically overcrowded, this is worth a try.

If none of this helps you, if at all possible, going at a different time can help. Mornings (especially weekend mornings) are classically empty, and of course during the day is the emptiest time of all.

> **I'm struggling with one of the lifts, and the supplementary videos don't help. What do I do?**

It's impossible to head off every possible issue anyone can have, which is where good trainers or coaches come in handy. But failing that, a community of people passionate about lifting, such as the Beasties community Discord for paying She's A Beast subscribers, is the next best thing (and I'm in there, too!). You can also try searching "[insert lift in question] mobility/exercises/stretches/mistakes," and you should get a bundle of resource articles and videos.

> **My gym only has squat/bench racks with fixed pegs, and none of them are the right height for me. What do I do?**

Too low is better than too high; you might have to almost do an extra rep to get the weight out of the pegs, but that's better than having to reach up too high or stand on your tippy toes. This scenario is not ideal, though, so if you want to continue training beyond LIFTOFF, you should look into finding a fully adjustable rack, whether that means asking your gym to get one or changing gyms.

I'm supposed to work out but feel like shit! What do I do?

I begrudge no one taking a bad day off. But also remember: 80% effort, or even 60%, is better than nothing. Barring an injury that needs to heal or one of the worst days of your life, you'll be set up better for getting back on track the next time if you do an admittedly shitty workout today than if you do no workout at all.

Many, or even most, days, you won't feel like the most powerful and confident person in the world. That's okay. Don't set that expectation. A lot of workouts can just be about checking the box and moving your pieces on the board forward. DO check in on your recovery and make sure you're not shortchanging yourself on rest or food.

Particularly in the interest of maintaining your habits, I'm a huge advocate of showing up, warming up, and doing whatever your first programmed movement is. If after that, you still feel like shit and would rather be anywhere else, leave. You did one lift! You will feel less bad when you pick up again than if you had done nothing.

If you earnestly want to complete the workout but just have no energy or enthusiasm, try shaving off 10% or 20% off your programmed working weights. This is NOT a failure; think of this workout as time to get your body moving, blood flowing, and to practice your form. You will never be able to get enough practicing your form. I've been doing this several years, and I'm still working on my form.

> **Lifting or even exercise in general feels uncomfortable for me; it hurts, or I just can't get over the embarrassment. What do I do?**

Barring and injury or debilitating soreness, let's talk about this. While I'm not God's gift to sports, I was an active kid and I played high school sports, and I often take for granted that I have a psychological background that reinforces physical activity: Exercise can cause (manageable!) amounts of physical discomfort and pain, but because it bonded me to my friends and siblings, and it gave me achievements and confidence in life, I am able to have positive associations with it. Others may feel a big fat nothing for exercise, or even have negative associations with it. And then on top of that, it IS a (manageable!) amount of physical discomfort and pain.

On the physical tip: All pain is not inherently bad (a good book about this is Ouch! Why Pain Hurts and Why it Doesn't Have To, by Kerr and Rodriguez). Don't take this too far, but a little pain can be good, and our bodies are built for the kind of overreaching that causes pain and progress. It may hurt, but you don't need to fear any hurt ever. Consider starting to work out as an experiment with exercise-specific discomfort that is ENTIRELY within your control. Try a little overreach here and there. Go as slowly as you need, but also strive to notice the payoffs. This is why taking notes and "weights go up" is important; you may even "see" progress in this way before you really "feel" it. You deserve those positive associations and validation, and you have to believe they can be built with practice.

On the emotional tip: I am not a psychologist, but the emotional/mental component of exercise is very real and I think affects more people than we realize. It also deserves to be taken seriously. If you have a goal or desire of learning to move and taking care of yourself but just can't get there, I very strongly suggest bringing it to a mental health professional. They CAN help with this.

■ I'm sore. What do I do?

As you start to lift, you might get sore or even experience the dreaded DOMS (delayed onset muscle soreness, which shows up between 24 and 48 hours after a workout). It's still okay to work out when you are sore, and it can even help lessen the soreness or shorten the overall time that you will feel sore.

If soreness is a frequent and bad problem for you, check in on your recovery. Soreness is very often the product of not eating enough, not sleeping enough, not drinking enough water, or external stress affecting all of these things.

If you thought you were eating enough, you might have been wrong. Lifting and building muscle requires fuel! This is not the time to restrict and diet.

If the soreness or pain gets worse as you warm up or start your working sets, stop. You might need to just take a day off. That's okay.

■ I hurt myself or have been sick! What do I do?

It can be hard to tell the difference between being sore and having an injury, like a strained muscle. But here is how to figure it out: Try to do your workout (gently!). If you feel less pain as you get warmer, it's probably just soreness. If the pain intensifies, you may be injured.

I can't tell you exactly how many workouts to skip, but try taking at least two or three workouts off (if the pain is local to one half your body, say your legs, try doing just your upper-body movements; again, 60% is better than nothing). Pay attention to how you feel.

If you end up taking a week or two off for whatever reason (illness, injury, inconvenience, sudden UFO abduction, etc.), when you go back, cut the weights you were working at by about 20 percent, and work your way back up according to the usual progression scheme.

And remember: Don't beat yourself up about this. "Progress" takes many forms, and you will always have to adapt to that. When you are injured, "progress" is "doing everything you can to help your injury heal as well as possible." Be gentle and patient with yourself physically and emotionally in these times!

■ I missed a day! What do I do?

If your schedule allows, you can take advantage of the two days off in a row in any given week and use one to get back on track. So if you typically go to the gym Monday-Wednesday-Friday, but you miss Monday, you do your Monday's workout Tuesday, Wednesday's on Thursday, Friday's on Saturday, then pick up again as normal the following Monday.

If you can only stick to your schedule, do the Monday workout you missed on Wednesday, which will just bump everything back a day (yes, this will throw off the spreadsheet a bit, but this is not a big deal).

And frankly, if you just have to go right ahead with the Wednesday workout, that's fine; it just means you're doing two of the same workout, 4-5 days apart. Strive to not make a habit of this, but it's not going to kill anyone.

■ **How will I know when I'm actually strong?**

I say this mostly in hopes it will bring you peace, but, as in all things, comparing yourself to others is usually not a fruitful activity. Honestly, speaking from experience, if you can handle a 45lb barbell with ease, like 95% of people's minds will be absolutely blown by that.

That said, you might want to know if you are taking advantage of all your potential! There is a thing called "strength standards" in lifting that will tell you roughly your total potential capacity based on your gender, height, weight, and age. These standards are notoriously tricky because a) there is not good data on women generally, and b) the data tends to be drawn from people who self-select into lifting, rather than a general population who happens to lift. Strength standards are nice to look at for a rough idea of where you're at, but nothing to ever feel bad about. There is one set of strength standards referenced on the Resources page.

▌ **I'm curious what my "one rep max" is, and/or I'm looking at some training programs that require me to know it, but I've only ever lifted weights for sets of five. How do I find this out?**

Other than trying it, there's no real way to know! You can use a purpose-built calculator to roughly guesstimate, but "maxing," as we say, is a skill that you build, and 1RM calculators are going to be assuming you have that skill. For instance, a 1RM calculator might say that if you can bench 80 pounds for 5 reps, you can bench 90 pounds for 1 rep. But if you've never done it before, you might only be able to bench 85 for one rep, while 90 pounds turns your arms into limp noodles. Testing your one-rep max will not create a helpful data point for a while still, though I strongly encourage pursuing it as a longer-term goal!

You can find a one-rep max calculators online, including ones that can take a number of reps you can do for a certain RPE, and then calculate for you how much weight to do for a different RPE or number of reps. Nifty! I would suggest using these calculators as a way of translating your current ability for a given number of reps (assume an RPE of 8) to other rep schemes over trying to convert it to a one-rep max and then back. For instance, according to this calculator, if you can bench 90 pounds for 5 reps at RPE 8, you can bench 81 pounds for 8 reps at RPE 8.

FURTHER CONSIDERATIONS

I do not claim to be an expert in the following areas, but if you are not the picture of youth (or maturity) or have disabilities or injuries, you might feel miffed by some parts of this text. But the world of strength training is more expansive and adaptable than you might think.

DISABILITIES AND INJURIES

Depending on your body, you might have factors that mitigate your ability to do the lifts as they're instructed here. This might include not being able to grip barbells; having limb asymmetries; or having prior injuries, like back problems.

Google won't give you medical answers. HOWEVER: it can be helpful in expanding your worldview of what is possible. Try searching for "powerlifter" or even "bodybuilder" + "[your disability or injury]", and there will very likely be someone out there who has found workarounds to being able to lift weights, or in the case of injury, has treated it and became more physically capable than they'd ever been before. This is not to suggest anyone with an injury or disability who doesn't "overcome" is a failure. It just may be more possible than you think.

In the vast majority of cases, doctors and medical professionals are overwhelmingly helpful and unfortunately underutilized, especially in the U.S. where basic medical care can be difficult to access and so expensive. But my one caveat here is that many doctors, especially older ones, cultivate a knee-jerk fear around heavy weights, and/or revolve their care ethos around "if it hurts, don't do that," which fails a lot of people when it comes to maintaining basic body functionality. For instance, if you have a bad back, lifting things improperly or even moving around might hurt very much. But learning to lift things *properly* and moving around more can be a total game changer, and it can turn out that the so-called bad back was not the barrier to fitness they or their doctor thought it was.

This doesn't mean "soldier on through a lifting program as if you have no ailments." But I'm begging you not to default to the presumption that because something hurts, your only choices are to avoid it or suffer. Sports medicine doctors or physical therapists can be very helpful at focusing on redeveloping functionality instead of telling you not to do what hurts.

AGE (YOUNG)

I can't in good conscience (or without liability) suggest that this program is a good idea for anyone under 18. But there are plenty of young people who do lift weights, and learning to do it properly from experts instead of from, say, your fellow bro on the football team who bounces the barbell off his sternum when he benches. There are also lots of kids who even compete in lifting weights; there are special considerations, but it's not impossible or really ill-advised at all. Look at the #kidswholift hashtag. Do me a personal favor and find a good coach first.

AGE (OLD)

At a point, our body's ability to build muscle starts to slow down. As we start to get up there in years, our capacity for building strength might not be what it once was. But that should be a different consideration from "feeling able to move," which strength training can really help with. As with the injuries point above, age should not be a default contraindication for lifting. If anything, you might benefit even more than a young person from doing what you can to preserve your muscle.

Please be careful of injuries, and check with your favorite medical professional that you are cleared for exercise (or, if you have health considerations, please strongly consider working with an informed trainer). But if you don't move well or aren't strong now, don't assume that means you can't learn. Look up the "masters" class of powerlifting competitions in the USPA and USAPL. Plenty of older people out there are still getting incredibly strong, and that could be you.

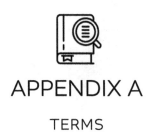

APPENDIX A

TERMS

To be honest, when I started lifting, I couldn't tell you with confidence the difference between a barbell and a dumbbell. So I'm going to teach you words now, and include some pictures. This is in alphabetical order.

BARBELLS

Here I am using a barbell with some plates loaded on it:

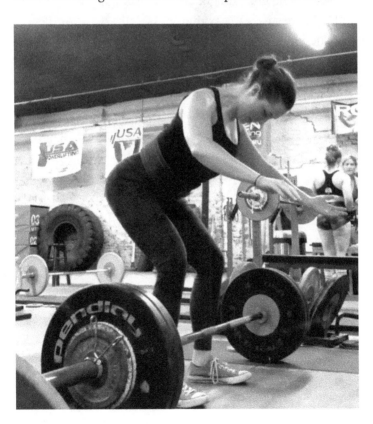

Barbells are used for all kinds of "compound movements," from squats to bench. They are not latched into a rack, and can be moved around freely. They weigh 45 pounds (or 20 kilograms), which is pretty heavy. There are barbells that weigh less or more than this, but they are pretty rare to find even within a specialty gym.

Barbells actually come in a great many varieties (Ohio Power Bar, Texas Power Bar, deadlift bar, Oly bar, etc.) and even different weights, but most barbells, especially at a generic gym, will be 45lbs. For the purposes of this program, you don't need to know anything more about barbells than "they are long and straight and you can put plates on both ends and they weigh 45 pounds."

The kind of barbell we are talking about is not "fixed barbells," which are shorter (3-4 feet long) and are a fixed amount of weight (10, 20, 50, 90lbs). While you actually *can* use them to help you bridge the gap between dumbbells and regular barbells, if your gym has them, the fact that that they aren't right-sized for a rack (see below) can work against you. For instance, you might be able to bench a 45lb barbell when it's safely in a rack, but trying to maneuver a 35lb fixed barbell into position over your head is an entire other story.

A barbell is also not a Smith machine (see "Rack").

BODY COMPOSITION/RECOMPOSITION

Broadly speaking, this is the types of mass your body is made up of, usually divided into your lean body mass (LBM) (organs, muscle tissue) and fat mass. At certain times or in certain states like when beginners start to lift, lifting weights can create a "recomposition" ("recomp") state, where bodies can lose body fat and gain muscle mass at the same time. This often, but not always, involves holding body weight constant and holding food intake at "maintenance" accordingly, i.e., not weight-loss-dieting.

CLIPS/COLLARS

Clips are bent springs with handles you can squeeze on one end to fit around the end of a barbell loaded with plates to keep the plates from sliding around. If your grip is too weak for the basic metal spring clips, I suggest investing a few dollars in a set of plastic barbell collars. You can keep them in your gym bag.

CUE

A mental trigger that is usually tied to a physical action. Cues are used to help develop good form in training, and are sometimes highly metaphorical, such as "tuck your shoulders to close your armpits, as if you are trying to prevent someone from tickling you." At the start, most compound lifts can feel like a lot of cues to think about at once. Ideally, eventually, cues develop into reflexes you don't have to think about so much.

COMPOUND LIFT

Movements that use multiple joint systems and muscle groups at once.

DUMBBELLS

This is a dumbbell:

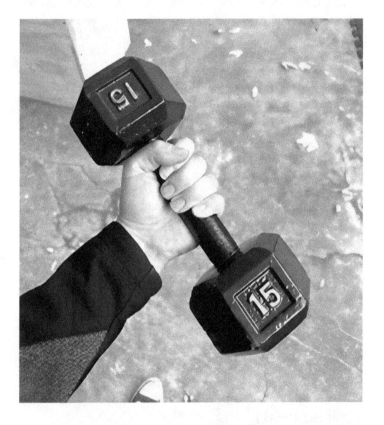

They are probably somewhat more familiar to you than barbells. When working with dumbbells, try to use two of the same weight and add them together. So for instance, if you want to start out squatting 20 pounds, use two 10lb dumbbells. When "weights go up" instructs you to add 2.5-5 pounds per lift, you are adding that to the total of your two dumbbells, not each dumbbell (though as always, you are always allowed to progress faster if you are able). If you squatted two 10lb dumbbells this session (20 pounds) you would squat 25 pounds (two 12.5lb dumbbells) next session.

"DEPTH" OR "ABOVE/BELOW PARALLEL" (AS IN SQUATS)

When you "hit depth," that means your squat is deep enough that the crease your hip makes where it folds is below the top of your knee, or "below parallel" (i.e. Your thighs are below parallel). Any higher than that is squatting "at" or "above parallel." Squatting to depth matters because your body uses different muscles once you reach below parallel, and it requires good, useful mobility that squatting above parallel does not.

FAIL/FAILURE/FAILING

You fail when you don't complete an intended lift. Failure is a core tenet of lifting. While failure is never the goal, if you never fail, you are probably not challenging yourself up to your potential. A great metaphor for life.

FORM/"GOOD FORM"

How you do a lift well. You can lift weights into the air really any way you want, but doing it "with good form" means you are doing it in a way that is maximally efficient for the way your body works, and is minimizing the potential for injury. Good form is generally easy-ish to learn but hard to master, but also, good form is not perfect form

FRACTIONAL PLATES

These are small, sub-5lb or 2.5kg plates, also known as "change plates" (I assume because they are kind of like change in your pocket). If your gym doesn't have them, it would be extremely worth the small amount of money it would cost to get the next size down from what your gym has and keep them in your bag or locker; 2.5-5lbs is not that much to carry, and being able to increment the weight is very helpful. If you don't want to do this, but your gym doesn't have plates that allow you to go up in increments smaller than 10lbs, you can use the progression scheme in the "What to do if you stall" section.

LINEAR PROGRESSION

Linear progression is a type of progressive overload where you add weights (or somehow increase intensity predictably) every session. Starter lifting programs are usually built around linear progression.

MAINTENANCE/MAINTAINING

"Maintenance" or "maintaining" is when you are not progressing or growing, but not backsliding either. This can be in terms of a specific metric (how much weight you are lifting, your body mass), or in all things. "Maintenance" in food is the rough amount required to hold one's body weight steady while they perform a certain amount of physical activity. Michael Phelps' maintenance food intake while he trains for the Olympics, for instance, is like 10,000 calories per day. For many of us, it's less than that.

MOBILITY

When a joint can move through its range of motion without pain or discomfort. Developing decent mobility is a goal of LIFTOFF; someone who can squat to depth or execute a hip hinge probably has good hip mobility. While some mobility is good, more mobility is not always better.

PLATES

Here I am using a barbell with some plates loaded on it:

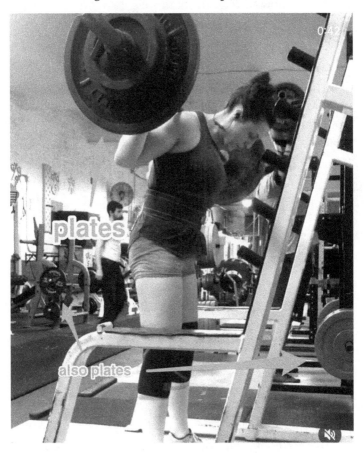

You may be most familiar with 45lb plates, but they can also come in 35lb, 25lb, 10lb, 5lb, 2.5lb, 1.25lb, and even smaller flavors.

"Bumper plates" are plates that are the same diameter as a standard 45lb plate, but weigh less (and are made of polyethylene or rubber).

Learning "plate math" is a whole thing, and someday will come extremely naturally to you. But you might be confused with how to refer to these weights: If you're lifting a 45lb barbell with a 5lb plate loaded on either end, are you lifting 5lbs? 10lbs? 55lbs?

The answer is you are lifting 55lbs; you always add all of the weight, including the barbell, together. When I say to "add 2.5lbs" to a lift when you are using a barbell, that would mean adding a 1.25lb plate to each end of the barbell. Weights should ALWAYS be loaded evenly on either side. You might load plates wrong by accident someday, because it happens to all of us, but do your best to load accurately and evenly.

PROGRESS/PROGRESSIVE OVERLOAD

"Progress" means, generally, "growth and change." Sometimes it means better form, better recovery, or simply not re-injuring your injury. Progress is always what we are shooting for in lifting (unless we are just maintaining). "Progressive overload" means each time you work out, you reach slightly beyond your comfortable capacity, allowing your body to build up your muscles slightly better than before (with food and rest). "Linear progression" is a type of progressive overload.

In this book, our form of progressive overload is to "weights go up," which means a) you add 2.5-5lbs to each lift every session, and b) you're not jumping into workouts with the aim of running yourself ragged and doing things that are too hard, such that you can't go up next time. You are creating the circumstances for sustainable growth, and that means challenging yourself, but *appropriately*, and taking care to recover from that challenge so you're ready for a slightly bigger challenge next time.

PULL

Any movement that involves "pulling" weights, such as lat pulldown, deadlifts, or rows.

PUSH

Any movement that involves "pushing" weights, such as squats, bench, overhead press.

RACK

The plates and barbell are used together in a rack, which ideally looks like this:

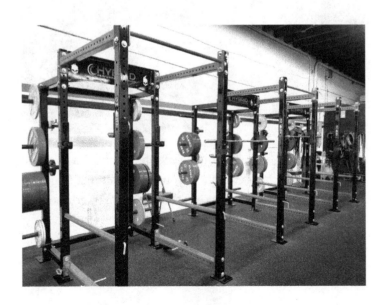

But may look like this or this if you are benching or squatting specifically:

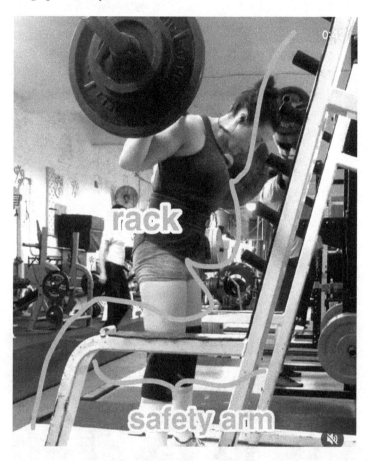

Ideally, any rack you use will have "safety arms" that can be adjusted to catch the weight if you overshoot and "fail," or have to drop it. Safety arms are those guys marked above.

If you are too short for the built-in safety arms in a squat rack, it's not ideal, but you can back all the way out of the rack so that you can get your full range of motion. Ideally, you should look for a gym with a power rack with fully adjustable arms and hooks, like the first picture.

If the rack looks very complex and the barbell is locked into it, such that you could not pick it up and carry it away with you: That's not a rack, that's a Smith machine. These are very common at chain gyms. Smith machines are more "machine" than "free weight," and don't work for our purposes for many reasons. In this program we use "free weights" so that our body has to support them in the same way it would support loads in the real world. Smith machines have their uses, but building functional strength is not really one of them for the purposes of LIFTOFF.

RANGE OF MOTION

How far your body can move in various directions. A contortionist who can sit on their own head has incredible range of spinal motion. Range of motion is often limited by mobility and flexibility, which are skills that are possible to develop. All the compound lifts in LIFTOFF require a good range of motion, which is a benefit in and of itself aside from strength.

RECOVERY

Recovery is essentially "anything you do outside the gym to support your training": eat, sleep, stretch, manage stress, walk. When your recovery is "good," it allows you to have good, fun, productive training sessions. When your recovery is "bad," it causes you to have painful, frustrating, annoying training sessions. While perfection is a myth, we strive for good recovery at all times: eating well and enough, sleeping well and enough, giving energy vampires the "sit, stay, go away" hand, and tending to any soreness with rest or gentle active recovery activities like walking or stretching. Good recovery is essential to the "weights go up" lifestyle and the overall constructive feedback loop of strength training; do not neglect it!

REP

One "rep" is one "repetition" of a movement. In the example of squats, when you sink down and come back up, that's one rep.

REST

The time between sets when you are not lifting, and you sit and do nothing. In LIFTOFF, this time ranges from 30 seconds to 2 minutes.

SET

A set starts when you pick a weight up intending to do a series of "reps," and ends when you finish the reps and put the weight down again. Between sets, when lifting weights, you rest anywhere from 30 seconds to a few minutes in this program.

SESSION

A session is one day of working out. In Phase One, there is only one type of session, repeated three times a week. In Phases Two and Three there are two types of sessions alternated throughout the weeks. When the program says to "add weight every session," that means if today, Monday, is Day A and you squat 40 pounds, the next time you do Day A on Friday (after your Day B on Wednesday) you squat 45 or even 50 pounds.

STALL

You stall when you aren't able to make progress in a given lift. For beginners, this is almost always the result of one or two things: insufficiently good form, and/or insufficiently good recovery. Barring those two issues, sometimes slowing or changing the progression scheme can help break the "plateau" where you are stalled (see the "What to do if you stall" section).

STRENGTH TRAINING, RESISTANCE TRAINING, WEIGHT LIFTING, WEIGHT TRAINING (AND BODYBUILDING)

All these terms (except bodybuilding) mean essentially the same thing: You are using weights to challenge your muscles and build strength. (The term "Resistance training" is most frequently used in scientific studies.) "Weightlifting" with no space usually refers to the sport of Olympic weightlifting, i.e. the "snatch" and "clean and jerk" movements. "Powerlifting" refers to the sport focused on the squat, bench, and deadlift movements. Powerlifting is the closest adjacent sport to the core of this program. "Strength training" technically means any training where strength is the goal. Strength training may be contrasted with "bodybuilding," where size or aesthetics is the goal. These two pursuits are often kept separate, but are loosely related; many lifters pursue both with "powerbuilding"-oriented programs. "Weight lifting" is the lifting of any weights, and could be any or all of these things.

WORKING WEIGHT/WORKING SETS

Usually this term is used in contrast to "warm-up weights" or "warm-up sets," but it's the amount of weight you are actually using for your sets. For instance, if you squatted 40 pounds last session for 5 sets of 5 reps, your working weight was 40 pounds. This session, you are adding 5 pounds, so your new working weight is 45 pounds, and your warm-up weights would be 22.5 pounds and 35 pounds.

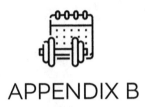

APPENDIX B

LIFTOFF PHASES ONE, TWO, AND THREE TEMPLATES

These are images for posterity.
Copy them into a notebook of your choice!

PHASE ONE, WEEKS 1-3

NOTE: You're using no weight / bodyweight / a light broom or swiffer or stick to practice movements with. Rest ~30 seconds between sets, remember to stay focused on practices, not speed or "working up a sweat."

*For body-weight squats, go to just below parallel, or as close to it as you can

**For incline push-ups, use a wall, back of a chair, coffee table; lower surfaces are harder, so if one surface gets too easy, move to a lower one

WEEK 1, 2, 3	DAY 1			
	EXERCISE	SETS	REPS	NOTES
	Overhead Press (OHP)	3	8	
	Bodyweight Squat*	3	10	
	Incline Pushup**	3	8	
	Hip Hinge	3	8	
	Bent Over Row	3	8	
	DAY 2			
	EXERCISE	SETS	REPS	NOTES
	Overhead Press (OHP)	3	8	
	Bodyweight Squat	3	10	
	Incline Pushup	3	8	
	Hip Hinge	3	8	
	Bent Over Row	3	8	
	DAY 3			
	EXERCISE	SETS	REPS	NOTES
	Overhead Press (OHP)	3	8	
	Bodyweight Squat	3	10	
	Incline Pushup	3	8	
	Hip Hinge	3	8	
	Bent Over Row	3	8	

PHASE TWO, WEEKS 4-8

*For dumbbell bench, if you don't have anything like a bench, substitute the "floor press" in the compendium.

**For lat pulldowns, if you aren't using a gym with a lat pulldown machine, but have a pullup bar, you can substitute a pullup progression (in the movement compendium). If you have neither, it's possible to hack together a pulldown setup from a resistance band and an anchor point, like a door. If you plan on progressing to phase 3 though, I strongly recommend starting to look around for a gym!

WEEK 4, 6, 8	DAY A			
	EXERCISE	SETS	REPS	LBS
	Dumbbell Squat	5	5	
	Dumbbell Bench*	5	5	
	Dumbbell Row	3	8	
	Notes			
	DAY B			
	EXERCISE	SETS	REPS	LBS
	Dumbbell RDL	5	5	
	Dumbbell OHP	3	5	
	Lat Pulldown**	3	8	
	Notes			
	DAY A			
	EXERCISE	SETS	REPS	LBS
	Dumbbell Squat	5	5	
	Dumbbell Bench	5	5	
	Dumbbell Row	3	8	
	Notes			

WEEK 5, 7	DAY B			
	EXERCISE	SETS	REPS	LBS
	Dumbbell RDL	5	5	
	Dumbbell OHP	3	5	
	Lat Pulldown	3	8	
	Notes			
	DAY A			
	EXERCISE	SETS	REPS	LBS
	Dumbbell Squat	5	5	
	Dumbbell Bench	5	5	
	Dumbbell Row	3	8	
	Notes			
	DAY B			
	EXERCISE	SETS	REPS	LBS
	Dumbbell RDL	5	5	
	Dumbbell OHP	3	5	
	Lat Pulldown	3	8	
	Notes			

PHASE THREE: WEEKS 9-12

NOTE: These are all barbell-based movements. If you don't have a barbell, plates, and a rack, thime to find a gym :) Record the weight you lift each session in the marked fields.

*For lat pulldowns, if you are able to, or prefer to do, a pull-up progression/variation(banded, negatives) go nuts. Just don't use the pullup machine

**For barbell squat, the variation you are doing is called "high bar" because it's easier to understand than other variations and is probably closest to what you already think a barbell squat is.

WEEK	DAY A			
9, 11	EXERCISE	SETS	REPS	LBS
	Barbell Deadlift	3	5	
	Overhead Press	3	5	
	Lat Pulldown*	3	8	
	Notes			

DAY B			
EXERCISE	SETS	REPS	LBS
Barbell Squat**	5	5	
Bench	5	5	
Bent Over Row	3	8	
Notes			

DAY A			
EXERCISE	SETS	REPS	LBS
Barbell Deadlift	3	5	
Overhead Press	3	5	
Lat Pulldown	3	8	
Notes			

WEEK 10, 12	DAY B			
	EXERCISE	SETS	REPS	LBS
	Barbell Squat	5	5	
	Bench	5	5	
	Bent Over Row	3	8	
	Notes			
	DAY A			
	EXERCISE	SETS	REPS	LBS
	Barbell Deadlift	3	5	
	Overhead Press	3	5	
	Lat Pulldown	3	8	
	Notes			
	DAY B			
	EXERCISE	SETS	REPS	LBS
	Barbell Squat	5	5	
	Bench	5	5	
	Bent Over Row	3	8	
	Notes			

CREDITS/SOURCES

Achieve Fitness, The 5 Minute Daily Mobility Routine, Jason and Lauren, March 28, 2021. Retrieved November 28, 2021.

Barbell Medicine, The Bench Press Prescription, March 22, 2018. Retrieved November 23, 2021.

Bret Contreras, Strong Curves, April 2, 2013.

Jennifer Case, Melissa Davis, Mike Israetel, Renaissance Woman, Renaissance Periodization.

Jordan Feigenbaum and Austin Baraki, The Beginner Prescription, Barbell Medicine, May 29, 2019. Retrieved November 23, 2021.

Molly Galbraith, GGS Secret to Mastering the Deadlift, Part 1, Girls Gone Strong. Retrieved November 23, 2021.

Molly Galbraith, GGS Secret to Mastering the Deadlift, Part 2, Girls Gone Strong. Retrieved November 23, 2021.

Eric Helms, Andy Morgan, and Andrea Valdez, The Muscle and Strength Pyramids: Training, 2018.

Eric Helms, Andy Morgan, and Andrea Valdez, The Muscle and Strength Pyramids: Nutrition, 2018.

Mike Israetel, James Hoffman, and Chad Wesley Smith, Scientific Principles of Strength Training, Renaissance Periodization.

Steve Kamb, Pull-up progression, Nerd Fitness, May 13, 2021. Retrieved November 23, 2021.

Steve Kamb, Beginner bodyweight workout, Nerd Fitness, February 3, 2021. Retrieved November 23, 2021.

Cody Lefever, GZCLP infographic, Say No to Bro Science. Retrieved November 23, 2021.
Mehdi, Stronglifts 5x5, Stronglifts. Retrieved November 23, 2021.
Michael Matthews, Thinner Leaner Stronger, January 6, 2014.
Michael Matthews, Beyond Bigger Leaner Stronger, August 20, 2014.
Mark Rippetoe and Andy Baker, Practical Programming for Strength Training, January 14, 2014.
Mark Rippetoe, Starting Strength: Basic Barbell Training, 3rd edition, November 11, 2011.
Alan Thrall, Stop deadlifting until you learn to do THIS, August 21, 2015. Retrieved November 23, 2021.
Reddit dumbbell stopgap, r/fitness. Sept 4, 2012. Retrieved November 23, 2021.
r/fitness basic beginner routine, r/fitness. Retrieved November 23, 2021.
Nutrition Wiki, r/XXFitness. Retrieved November 23, 2021.
Optimal Daily Protein Intake Guide, Examine.com, Sept 20, 2021. Retrieved November 23, 2021.
Power rack image by George Pagan III.

ACKNOWLEDGEMENTS

A very warm thank you to all the members of the She's A Beast community who were so kind to beta-test this program before its launch. Thank you to the coaches of Murder of Crows Barbell, Sean Collins, Matt Cronin, and Jean LaGuerre Jr., who taught me many things about strength that books could never. Special thanks to Kelsey McKinney, Libby Watson, Troy Coll, Josh Gondelman, and Casey Newton, all of whom helped with tasks ranging from reading my drafts to yelling at me vigorously to believe in myself. A very special thanks to Seamus McKiernan, whose kindness, love, enthusiasm, and insight defy words.

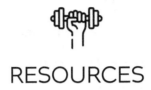

RESOURCES

These are external resources listed in the book, in alphabetical order.

Cronometer https://cronometer.com/

Eat This Much https://www.eatthismuch.com/

ExRx Strength Standards https://exrx.net/Testing/WeightLifting/StrengthStandards

FitMenCook https://fitmencook.com/

GZCLP https://thefitness.wiki/routines/gzclp/

MealPrepManual https://mealprepmanual.com/

MyFitnessPal https://www.myfitnesspal.com/

MacroFactor https://macrofactorapp.com/bmr-calculator/

The She's A Beast Pull-Up Progression https://store.shesabeast.co/products/liftoff-couch-to-barbell-pull-up-progression

Renaissance Diet 2.0, RP Strength https://rpstrength.com/products/rp-diet-book-v2

Renaissance Woman, RP Strength https://rpstrength.com/products/rp-female-book

She's A Beast https://www.shesabeast.co/

She's A Beast review of Intermediate programs, part one https://www.shesabeast.co/all-the-directions-you-can-go-with/

And part two https://www.shesabeast.co/intermediate-programs-part-two-rise-sbtd-momentum-review/

Tactical Barbell https://www.tacticalbarbell.com/

XXFitness Nutrition Wiki https://www.reddit.com/r/xxfitness/wiki/nutrition/

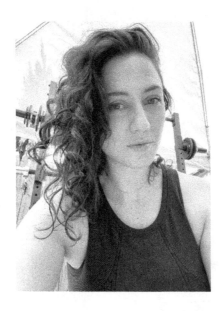

AUTHOR BIO

Casey Johnston has been bringing the joys of lifting weights to the people since 2016 with her beloved health advice column, Ask A Swole Woman, which published at outlets included The Hairpin, VICE, and Self. Casey has worked for over a decade as a science and tech journalist and editor, and has written for outlets including the New York Times, the New Yorker, The Awl, and Hazlitt. She loves lifting. She looOOooves lifting. Because of that, she has written a newsletter since 2021 called She's A Beast, about getting stronger mentally, emotionally, and physically.

She holds a bachelor's degree in applied physics from the Columbia University engineering school, and an NASM certification in personal training.

www.ingramcontent.com/pod-product-compliance
Lightning Source LLC
LaVergne TN
LVHW091949180725
816540LV00022B/135